E-Z A B

E-Z A B GEEZ

ARTERIAL BLOOD GASES

Written and Illustrated by
Gregory L. Culver, M.D., FAAFP

VANTAGE PRESS
New York

FIRST EDITION

Published by Vantage Press, Inc.
516 West 34th Street, New York, New York 10001

Manufactured in the United States of America
ISBN: 0-533-12697-5

Library of Congress Catalog Card No.: 98-90061

0 9 8 7 6 5 4 3 2

To my
Wife,
Rozzmerri
the best Medical Technologist,
with supreme inspiration . . .
gentle critique . . .
heartfelt support . . .
and red hair

Contents

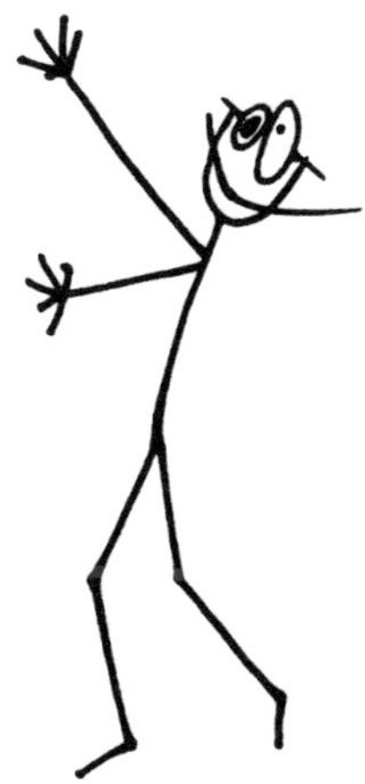

Preface

Arterial Blood Gases (ABG's) tell us the partial pressure of each essential gas, at the moment of drawing the sample, in the oxygenated arterial blood of the patient's vascular system. This is helpful information for evaluating the status of cardiac, pulmonary, ventilated, and other critically ill patients. The acid-base balance is intricately related to this "gas status." ABG's may be indicated whenever respiratory, cardiac, renal, or pH concerns are present. They are extremely valuable in managing a patient through a "code arrest." But . . . gases blow.

As advertised, medical school was the ultimate challenge for me. I was in "Special Ed." While the other students delved into pathophysiology and pharmacology, we were taking field trips to the nursing home to paint pumpkins. Perhaps that was, in part, why I was so baffled one night when an ICU nurse first bestowed upon me a cascade of jumbled numbers called "A B GEEZ." Try as I would, for years understanding was slow to dawn. But it did. Presented in this book is a simple (trust me) method of thoroughly understanding blood gases. Whoever you are, MD, DO, MS, RN, NS, LPN, EMT, PA, NP, ACLS, JD, or whatever other fancy initials, this method should serve you well.

For completeness I have included a first chapter on the clinical drawing of blood gases. Chapter IV presents a systematic approach to reading any set of blood gases. It is my own unique method. One doesn't need to mathematically verify ABG findings to read them accurately, so the reader may skip chapter V. However, the mathematics do add a certain confidence and reliability to the interpretation.

The reader will note that I have taken the liberty of oversimplifying some very complex concepts in the writing of this book. This was not done to play down the importance of these intricate issues. Rather, I have striven to present a learnable method for ABG analysis to virtually any interested reader. Please pardon detailed accuracy in some explanations to fully appreciate a viewpoint that is easier to remember and therefore learn.

In one lesson the reader can be prepared to efficiently draw and consistently interpret arterial blood gases correctly. If you find this book too difficult, do what I did—spit out your gum.

E-Z A B GEEZ

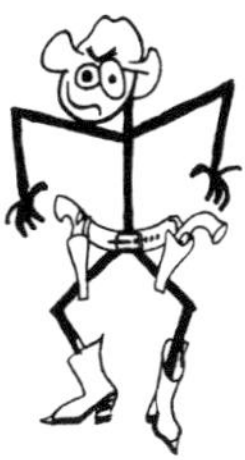

I

THE DRAW

A. Materials

First you'll need a patient. The **indications** for ABG's are varied. Basically anyone needing evaluation of blood gas partial pressures or acid-base balance is a candidate. Cardiac and respiratory patients are common targets. Likewise, any "code-arrest" patient will do.

The patient need not be alive. Dead (or mostly dead) patients can usually be drawn quite nicely as long as **CPR** is providing an adequate pulse. But remember, "pulse" does not necessarily equate to "flow." Imagine a garden hose with the faucet on and the sprayer end off. Even though there is no flow of water in the hose, stomping on one end will provide a "pulse" to a person holding the far end of the hose. The blood flow in a code arrest patient will be less than optimal. However, if a pulse is palpable, an ABG specimen syringe can usually be filled. If the pulse is poor . . . bring a book. If a pulse is not palpable, do not attempt an arterial stick.

Most hospitals now have nifty little pre-packaged

ABG **draw kits.** The needle is already mounted, but it helps to twist it down firmly to ensure that the Leur-lock is tight. The syringe is a "vented" type, i.e., the plunger is pulled back to the desired amount of specimen in milliliters before the draw. During the draw, the syringe is filled by arterial pressure plus capillary action without any further movement of the plunger. The air in the specimen portion of the syringe is vented out as it is replaced by rising blood. The packages may also include cute little silicon cubes to safely embed the needle after the draw. Use only one hand—do not hold the "cube" in a free hand (yours or otherwise). "Inadvertent inoculation" sparks reams of paperwork and a real risk of bad bugs.

Hand condoms are likewise a must. **Gloves,** while not bullet-proof, keep fingers from getting "red wet." Remember the Rule of Universal Precautions: "If it's wet and it ain't yours, don't touch it." Use gloves.

You will need an **antiseptic** skin prep. At best, alcohol is bacteriostatic, not bactericidal. Reference to alcohol should be reserved for the popular bar drinks. Use something else. My favorite anti-lawyer sauce is Betadine (Providone Iodine).

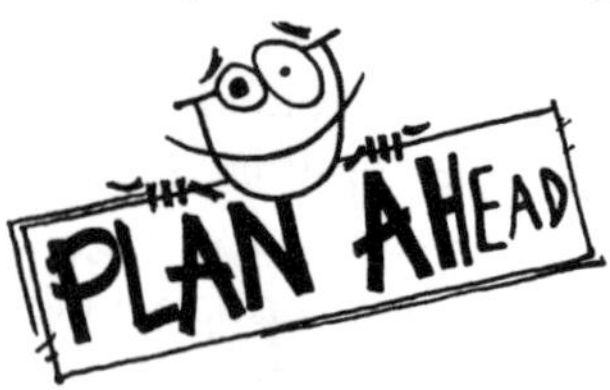

After the draw, you will need to cover the puncture site and hold pressure for at least two minutes to avoid bleeding. A "two-by-two" gauze folded into fourths works well as a pressure dressing. I like to hold it in place with a cloth **Band-aid,** but any approved hospital tape (legalized duct tape) will do just fine. It should be at least as wide as the folded gauze for proper pressure. I press through the dressing for two minutes, then leave it in place. You may find a cute nearby nurse to hold two minutes of pressure for you. If you subscribe to the adage that, "No bleeding is truly significant until you can hear it," you may even have the patients hold their own pressure. However, once you have a hematomato the size of a gorilla's left testicle, you will probably hold your own for two minutes.

Lastly, if it will be fifteen minutes or more until the sample is run in the lab, you will want to "**ice**" the specimen. I like to stuff the sample (needle down) into a patient's bedside ice pitcher.

Let's talk technique. . . .

B. Arterial Choice

The most common artery for an ABG draw ("arterial stick") is the radial. It's chosen in most non-emergent situations. The femoral is used commonly in a code when the arms are poorly accessible by people starting IV's, doing chest compressions, monitoring, defibrillating, and weeping. Another commonly used artery in routine draws is the brachial. With the widespread fear that the femoral stick hurts more and is more likely to become infected, the brachial is chosen when the radial is either not wise (see the Allen Test ahead) or is unsuccessful. In a pinch, any peripheral artery can be fair game. (But, contrary to what one of my medical students thought, retinal and dorsal penile attempts during a code are NOT funny.)

C. Procedure

I'll cover two techniques for arterial stick. They are the radial and femoral techniques. Between the two you'll be able to apply the principles to draw any artery.

The **radial artery** is easily located in the radial groove running longitudinally on the superior aspect of the distal anterior forearm just superior to the flexor carpi radialis tendon. (Just take the pulse at the wrist like they do on TV.) The ulnar artery can frequently be palpated in its corresponding location parallel to the radial artery on the inferior aspect of the wrist. The two anastomose in the hand to form the palmar arches.

Before attempting a radial draw, ensure that the ulnar artery is patent with the **Allen Test.** This ensures that the hand will not necrose and fall off if you damage or occlude the radial during the procedure. Have the patient make a tight fist with the back of the hand and wrist on a firm flat surface. Using your thumb and index finger, tightly occlude the radial and ulnar arteries with downward pressure. Have the patient open his or her hand while noting the palm is somewhat pale. Remove the occlusion from the ulnar artery and observe the palm to "flush." This shows patency of the ulnar artery if the hand flushes in under five seconds. You can safely proceed with a radial stick. On occasion, especially with patients having peripheral vascular disease, the Allen Test will not flush the palm until the radial is released. Proceeding with radial stick may compromise the circulation to the hand. Reevaluate the risk to benefit ratio and consider another site. Most of my patients have two arms.

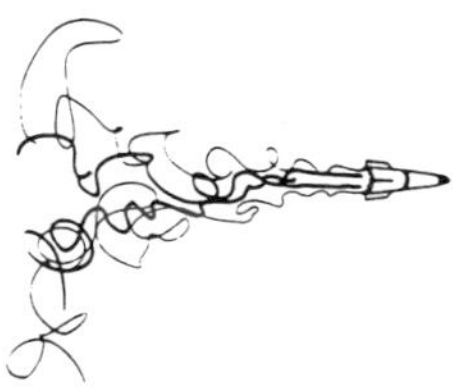

My nickname in medical school was "Torpedo." I was tall and slender. It was said I was incapable of thinking and had somewhat of a single-mindedness in attitude. I would launch off on a task at high speed in a single direction without wavering. I was capable of causing insurmountable damage in a matter of seconds. Not true. I was not tall at all. As you set out to stab needles into someone's artery for the first time, it's a good idea to bring along an instructor. Most medical technologists are quite eager to help.

Explain to the patient that arteries are muscular and highly innervated (supplied with nerves). Compared to the usual venous draw that they are accustomed to, the arterial stick will probably be more painful. (Now they won't think your technique simply stinks!)

Don your gloves. Expose the patients wrist. Supinate the forearm (turn the hand "palms up" like holding a bowl of hot chicken "sup"). I like to hyperextend the hand over the cute little Kleenex box found on every patient's bedside stand. Palpate the radial pulse with BOTH your index and middle fingertips spread 1 cm apart along the length of the artery as close to the wrist as possible. It is important to find the pulse with BOTH fingertips. Gently "rock" pressure back and forth between the fingers and LOOK at the 1 cm space between them. Picture the artery and imagine its course running below BOTH your fingers. The target is between your fingers. The needle will be placed here. Rock pressure to the most distal fingertip and ease off pressure on the proximal fingertip. This will distend the artery between the fingers to assist in filling the specimen syringe.

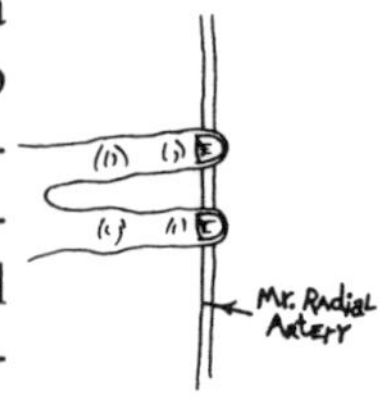

Quickly wipe antiseptic between your fingers on the skin of the wrist overlying the artery without moving your two fingers that are palpating the artery. Grasp the syringe in your free hand and turn the bevel on the needle to face proximally, i.e., the "hole" in the needle tip should point "upstream."

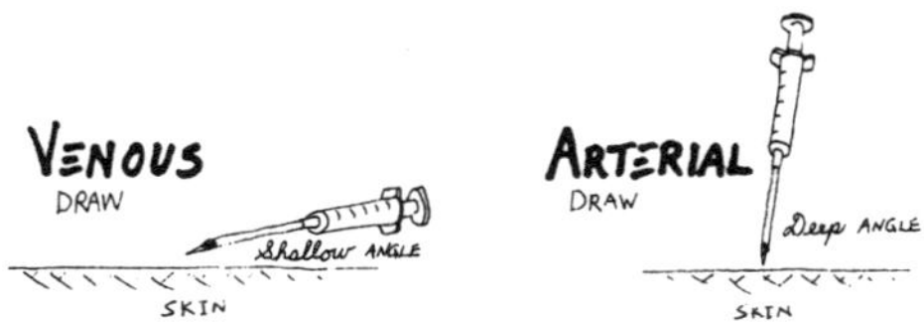

Hold the syringe "high." In a venous draw, the needle-to-skin angle of entry is shallow. In an arterial draw the angle is deep—nearly vertical. Aim at the artery between your fingers. In one quick jab, pierce the skin, and attempt to enter it. At any time you get a sudden flash of blood— FREEZE—and allow the syringe to fill.

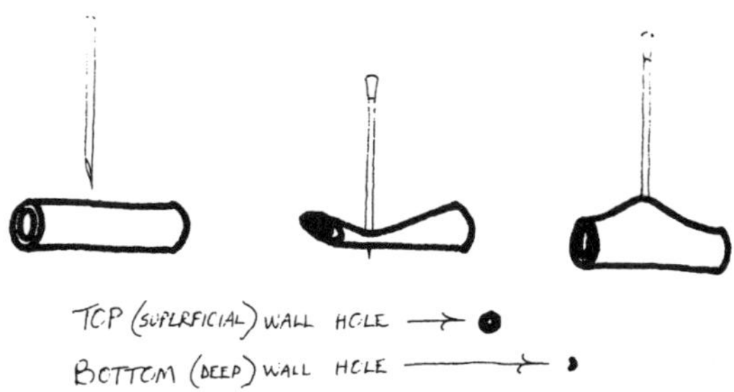

Let's pause a moment to talk mechanics. There is a superficial and deep wall of the artery. If your aim has been true, you've just put a hole in both and the walls have nearly collapsed together. The needle may not fill.

But the hole in the superficial wall is big. It's a full diameter of the needle shaft. The longitudinal and circular muscle layers in the wall of the artery are tight around it. Therefore, the superficial wall grasps the needle. The deep wall has a smaller slitlike hole made by only the tip of the hypodermic needle. Only the tip of the needle is imbedded here and the "grasp" is loose. The tip can dislodge easily.

If initially the syringe does not begin filling, give a quick, but slight, upward pull. Then allow the needle to relax downward. This "tents" the superficial wall upward, but allows the deep wall to stay deep, thus "opening" the lumen of the artery. Repeat this **quick but slight upward pull followed by relaxation back downward** until either the syringe begins to fill or the needle is withdrawn from the skin. If at any time filling begins, FREEZE and allow the syringe to fill. If the needle is fully withdrawn, redirect it once either medially or laterally and repeat the initial thrust. Repeat the withdrawal by multiple rapid, but limited upward thrusts.

Once filling begins, allow the syringe to fill completely. There must be no air bubbles. Remove the needle and seal the syringe into the silicon cube or capping device provided. See that the tube is rolled and "agitated" to fully dissolve the anticoagulation pellet found in the syringe. This avoids clotting. Hold direct firm pressure for two minutes.

If you fail to fill the syringe on the "second pass,"

quickly, find a way to place the blame on the nearest nurse, then proceed onto a new site. It's no good to persist with a multitude of attempts on a single artery. I have seen too many wrists that look like they were attacked by rabid sewing machines. This is where arterial occlusion complications are born. Limit yourself to two passes per artery.

The **femoral artery** is found in the groin. Find the inguinal ligament. Don't be fooled by the inguinal fold. The fold is the crease between the abdominal fat pad and the top of the leg. It has no predictable relationship

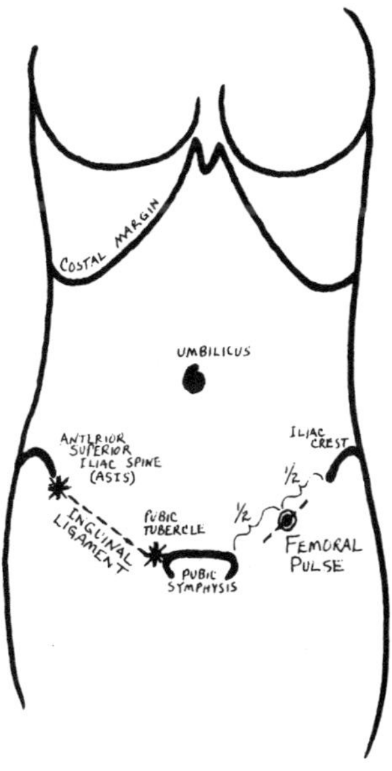

to the inguinal ligament. It will vary according to the degree of adiposal panniculus (degree of obesity). Find the inguinal ligament by identifying a line from the anterior superior iliac spine to the pubic tubercle. The ASIS is the forwardmost bump on the iliac crest (hip bones). The tubercle is the bump on the far lateral aspect of the pubic symphysis. Place a finger on both. Imagine a line between the two. This is the tract of the inguinal ligament. Envision the midpoint. Palpation here will reveal the femoral pulse.

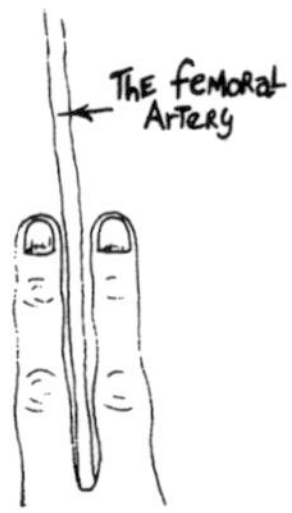

The anatomy of the structures in the femoral neurovascular bundle is easily remembered by the mnemonic "NAVY." In the human crotch, from the lateral to medial aspect, one finds the femoral nerve, artery, then vein. (The "Y" is the crotch.) During an arterial stick in the groin, avoid inadvertently passing medially into the femoral vein. ABG's on blue blood test out funny if you think it's red stuff. Unlike the radial draw, when finding the femoral pulse, keep your fingertips together over the artery. Feel it with both fingertips of your index and long finger. Then rotate your hand 90

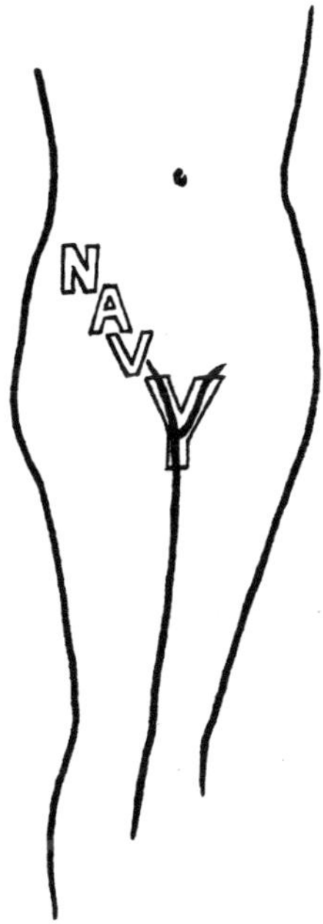

degrees and slightly separate your fingers until you can feel the pulse on the insides of both fingertips. The artery now runs in the same direction as the long axis of your fingers (and between them). Be sure to keep your fingers close enough together to maintain the pulse palpable in BOTH fingers.

Wipe antiseptic between your fingers without moving them. Proceed on with the arterial stick exactly as under the radial draw.

Between the radial and the femoral techniques, no

peripheral artery should be safe from your clinical probings.

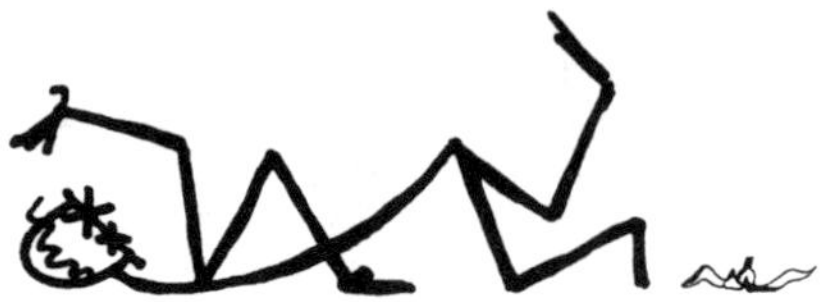

D. Pitfalls

Several screw-ups can occur in the collection of arterial blood gases. The most common problems are outlined here.

An inadvertent **venous draw** can be very misleading to the practitioner caring for a patient. The oxygenation is poor and carbon dioxide content high in a venous sample. Keep your fingers on the pulse. At no time should you attempt an arterial stick without a palpable pulse. In both techniques you should have the pulse in BOTH fingertips. Watch the filling of the syringe. You can see a slight "ebb and flow" filling pattern with each pulse on most arterial entries. Avoid "going medial" on a femoral draw. Don't rely on the "color" of the blood to determine an inadvertent venous draw—it is rarely accurate.

A neat trick to verify that you do in fact have a true arterial sample is to look at the O_2 SATURATION. This value tells the percent of hemoglobin that is carrying oxygen molecules. If it is greater than 75%, you can rest assured that you have an arterial draw since venous blood will always be less than 75%. However, if O_2 SAT is below 75%, you can NOT conclude that you have a venous sample. In this case, it may be arterial with the patient having severe respiratory trouble and subsequent crap for oxygenation.

Another common mistake is to allow **air bubbles** to remain in the specimen syringe at completion of the draw. Once you strike oil—FREEZE! Allow the syringe to fill COMPLETELY. If filling stops before it is full, GENTLY and steadily withdraw the needle upward. Unlike the "quick but slight upward pull followed by relaxation back downward" maneuver used to *acquire* the arterial fill, here the lumen has already been found. When lost, draw back slowly and steadily. If filling resumes—FREEZE. If not, continue on out from the skin. If at the end of any draw there are still air bubbles, invert the syringe to a "needle up" position and push in the plunger of the syringe until all the air is evacuated. If the sample isn't of a sufficient volume, you'll know it soon enough from the laboratory. If you leave air in the sample, the arterial gases will continue to exchange with the air bubble and render the results invalid (or worse— misleading).

Avoid **a clotted sample.** Once the blood is obtained and the needle secured, hold the syringe in both hands in a "praying" fashion. Roll it. Another agitation technique is to "topple" the syringe end over end several times. The object is to dissolve and mix the anticoagulation pellet completely throughout the blood sample. A clotted sample is a complete waste. It cannot be run through the analyzer. If partially clotted, it will give inaccurate partial pressures.

Dropping the syringe and shattering it nine ways to hell on the floor is not common, but is a favorite of mine. This maneuver should probably be avoided, especially by medical students. Their lives are already sufficiently complicated.

If the **sample warms,** the blood gases will shift out of solution and give inaccurate readings. Label the specimen with the patient's name, hospital number, time of draw, and what oxygen (if any) was being administered to the patient at the time of the draw. If more than fifteen minutes are likely to elapse before the sample is run, it must be iced.

An arterial embolus into the leg is rare from a femoral draw and unlikely in a brachial. The more distal the draw, the more severe an **arterial complication** will be. Radial, then, is the most commonly complicated and the most severe. Limit yourself to two attempts at any arterial site. Always perform and document the Allen Test before attempting a radial stick. In all testing, weigh the possibility of complication against the potential benefit of the information you will obtain by performing the study. Black dead hands are a bummer.

With practice you'll soon be drawing ABG's slicker than hot chicken fat on a stuck doorknob. The lab will fire back piles of numbers. Let's turn to making sense out of 'em!

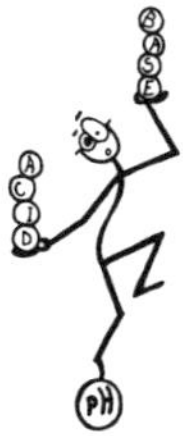

II

BALANCING ACT

The human body maintains itself within a realm of normalcy in all parameters. From blood pressure control to body temperature regulation, the body protects this range of norm. This feature is known as **homeostasis.**

Acid-base balance is one of the variables held within a narrow window by homeostasis. Outside this window the blood becomes too acidic or too basic. Having blood that is too acidic is called **acidemia**—NOT to be confused with the term "acidosis" covered later. Having blood that is too basic or alkaline is called **alkalemia**—NOT to be confused with the term "alkalosis" covered later.

So, who cares?!? Very few tissues, organs, or systems work well in extremes of acid-base imbalance. For example, neurotransmission is poor in alkalemic states (thus the parethesias of hyperventilation) and cerebral edema can occur when severe. Acidemic hearts are very prone to dyshythmias and are resistant to defibrillation. **Acid-base balance,** the maintenance of **proper oxygenation,** and the **elimination of carbon dioxide** from the body are all imperative and all closely linked.

The body uses **buffering systems** to maintain acid-base balance. There are many—some minor and a few major. The large proteins in the serum are minor contributors. Hemoglobin is a complex molecule capable of some buffering. Hemoglobin and other large proteins buffer by virtue of accepting or deferring free hydrogen ions. But, for truly potent pH balance, a system would need to go to the source and actually change the amount of acid or base. These would be the major systems. There are two. They are the **renal** and **respiratory** systems. Let's compare and contrast the two.

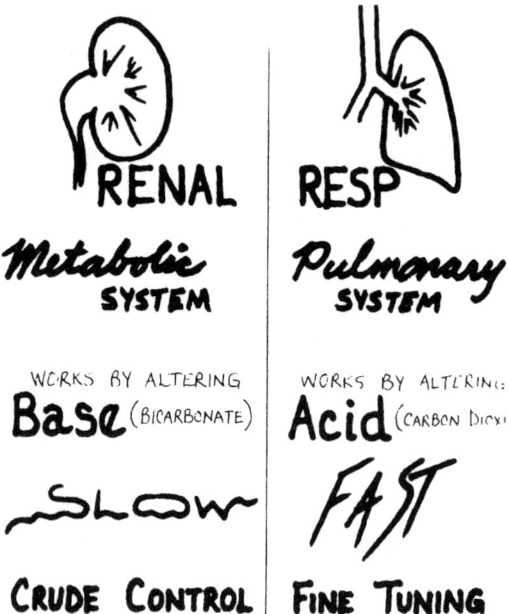

The **RENAL** component of pH balance is the **metabolic system.** It influences pH by **altering base** (bicarbonate to be exact). It is a **slow** system and offers only **crude control.** By remembering that this system works more slowly over time, one can frequently infer how long an aberration has been present.

The **RESPIRATORY** component of acid-base balance, carried out by the **pulmonary system,** influences pH by **altering acid.** The acid it regulates is carbon dioxide. The understanding that CO_2 is an acid is paramount to interpreting ABG's. The respiratory system acts very **quickly** and offers "**fine tuning**" compared to the renal system's slow crude control.

Carbon dioxide reacts with water to form carbonic acid—a mediary on the way to dissociation into bicarbonate and free hydrogen ion. For those of you who like chemistry, the formula is:

$$CO_2 + H_2O \rightleftharpoons H_2CO_3 \rightleftharpoons HCO_3^- + H^+$$

CARBONIC ACID

I personally detest chemistry. One of the most common problems I've seen folks have in ABG interpretation stems from their failure to remember that carbon dioxide acts as an acid. Sock this tidbit away: **"CO_2 is an acid!"**

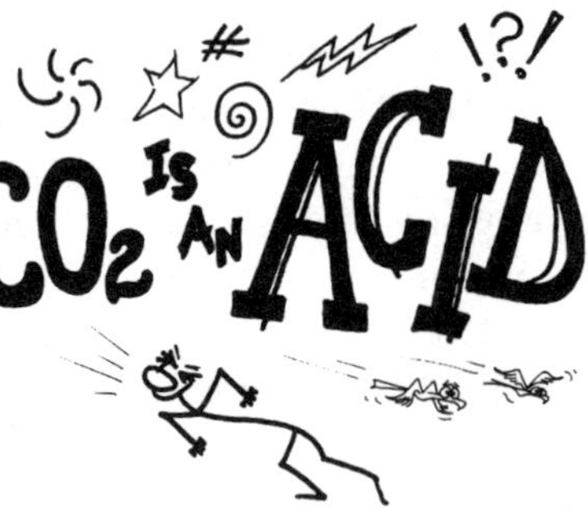

I would hate to insult your intelligence, but something must be solid here. To the reader already clear on this point, I regret the intrusion. Acid-base balance is measured in **pH.** A normal pH is 7.40, with a normal range of 7.35 to 7.45. As the body becomes ACIDEMIC, the pH DROPS to a lower value. As the body becomes ALKALEMIC, the pH RISES to a higher pH. Enough said.

The suffix "-emia" means "the blood overall." Acidemia means the blood overall is too acidic. Alkalemia means overall the blood is too basic. The suffix "-osis" refers to a diagnosis. Each system can contribute its part. There can be a respiratory acidosis or alkalosis. There can be a metabolic acidosis or alkalosis. There can be combinations of the two systems. Either the respiratory system or metabolic system (or both) may be normal. An alteration in one system is frequently "compensated" by the other system. This represents an attempt to "correct" the primary problem (i.e., recover homeostasis). There are, therefore, nine possibilities:

1. Normal RESPIRATORY, Normal METABOLIC } NORMAL ACID BASE BALANCE
2. "Pure" RESP ACIDOSIS (Metabolic normal)
3. "Pure" RESP ALKALOSIS (Metabolic normal)
4. "Pure METAB ACIDOSIS (Respiratory normal)
5. "Pure" METAB ALKALOSIS (Respiratory normal)

6. RESP ACID, METAB ACID } "COMBINED ACIDOSIS"
7. RESP ALK, METAB ALK } "COMBINED ALKALOSIS"

} These two are the "combined" states. In each of these two, the alteration in one system is being added to by the same type of alteration in the other system.

8. RESP ACID, METAB ALK
9. RESP ALK, METAB ACID

} These last two are the "compensating" states. In each of these two, the alteration in one system leads to an attempt in the other system to correct it.

Before we dive into the reading of a set of ABG's, let's zoom through a few frequently seen scenarios.

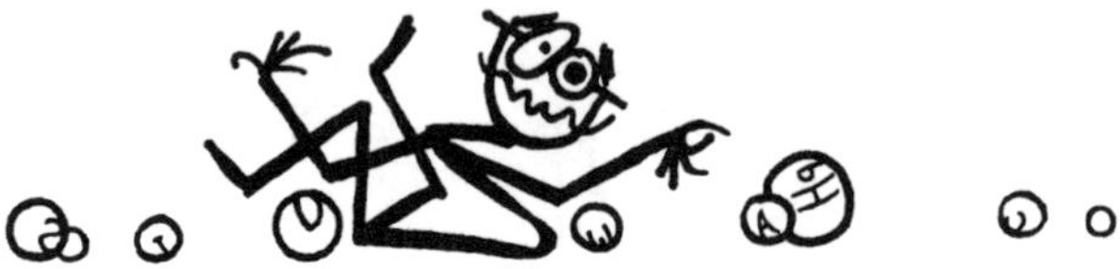

III

COMMON SCENES

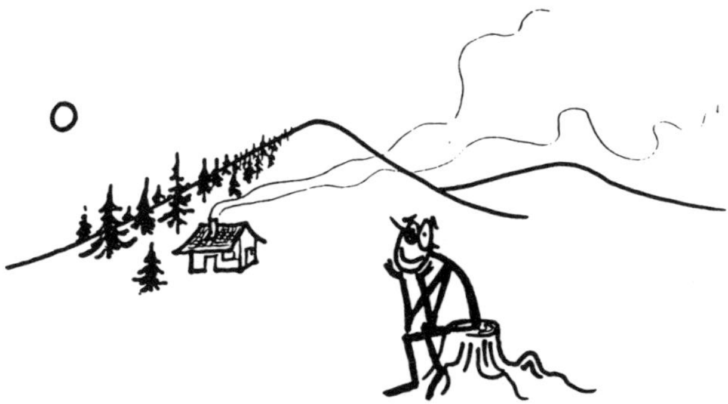

A. Hyperventilation

When a normal person holds their breath, the partial pressure of carbon dioxide (pCO_2) climbs. This is the normal stimulus for respiratory drive. Surprise! The level of oxygen in the arterial blood (measured as pO_2) has little to do with respiratory drive. A normal person therefore runs on a so-called "hypercarbic drive." It's not the "low oxygen" that makes us want to breathe, it's the high carbon dioxide. This is in contrast to a "chronic lung" patient (see COPD/Emphysema below).

There's more. If the pCO_2 falls too LOW, it ALSO is a stimulus to breathe, i.e., hypocarbia drives respiration as well. Therefore, it is more of an *imbalance* of CO_2 than a simple *elevation* of CO_2 that provokes breathing.

Having a low pCO_2 provoke the respiratory drive is out of the norm. But, it *is* the basis of hyperventilation syndrome. Anytime the "minute volume" of respirations (the volume of air in and out of the lungs in one minute) climbs high enough to "blow off" too much CO_2, hyperventilation can ensue. The pCO_2 falls below normal. Remember that "CO_2 is an acid." With this loss of acid, a respiratory alkalosis occurs. The low pCO_2 stimulates the respiratory drive. Paradoxically the patient feels dyspneic and breathing effort increases. Subsequently more CO_2 is blown off and the problem goes on to propagate itself in a positive feedback loop.

The determinate here is minute volume—not simple respiratory rate. One can breathe faster or deeper or both to increase minute volume and precipitate hyperventilation. The syndrome is frequently seen in athletes, asthmatics, public speakers, clergy, long-winded politicians, and other anxious people. It is also commonly seen in patients with acute severe pain from any cause. Angry hospital administrators have been known to severely hyperventilate while negotiating physician salaries.

Hyperventilation can terribly confuse a clinical history. The signs and symptoms can be misleading.

Learn to recognize the syndrome. Watch for dyspnea, tachypnea, chest discomfort, tachycardia, diaphoresis, pallor, tremor, circumoral numbness, face/hand numbness, "tingling," "weak knees," "butterflies in the stomach," nausea, dry mouth and sweaty palms. Notice that many findings represent sympathetic nervous system outflow symptoms.

Hyperventilation syndrome manifested as respiratory alkalosis can be seen alone or in combination with other acid-base pathology. If no other pathology is present, the ABG's will show a pure respiratory alkalosis with excellent oxygenation.

B. Pulmonary Embolus

When a blood clot travels into the right heart and is tossed out into the pulmonary vasculature, it can lodge in the arterial tree to cause a pulmonary embolus. Air will get to that segment of the lung, but no gas exchange will occur because blood cannot get into the area beyond the clot.

The patient classically has a feeling of impending doom with something terribly wrong in the chest. Dyspnea is nearly universal and chest pain common. Expect to see all the signs and symptoms of hyperventilation including respiratory alkalosis.

A quick point here. CO_2 diffuses across alveolar membranes much faster and easier than O_2. This explains how in pulmonary embolus, hyperventilation blows down CO_2 causing respiratory alkalosis even with part of the lung out of order. However, with this non-participating piece of lung, enough oxygen can not be taken up through the remaining lung and so some degree of hypoxia is almost always seen (on room air testing). Bronchoconstriction may play a part as well.

In a previously healthy patient, a sudden pulmonary embolus will usually show a pure respiratory alkalosis. However, unlike a simple hyperventilation syndrome in which oxygenation is great, a pulmonary embolus will tend to show hypoxia.

C. COPD/Emphysemia

Chronic lung disease encompasses **Chronic Obstructive Pulmonary Disease (COPD)** in which there is air trapping/hyperinflation of the lungs with obstruction of exhalation and **Emphysema** in which alveolar walls are destroyed leading to less surface area for gas exchange. Both are usually found in combination and are nearly always a consequence of long- term cigarette smoking. “Sucking butts” remains a great national pastime and should provide you with plenty of practice in ABG’s for years to come.

As the lungs are slowly ruined in chronic lung disease, two things gradually happen. The pCO_2 climbs and the pO_2 drops. Recall that the normal respiratory stimulus is a "hypercarbic drive." In chronic lung disease, the chronically high pCO_2 causes the respiratory center to begin IGNORING high pCO_2 as a stimulus to breathe. Gradually more attention is paid to the low oxygen stimulus and these patients evolve into a "hypoxic drive." This explains the occasional COPD/Emphysema patient who goes into respiratory arrest when given full flow oxygen. The respiratory drive is simply turned off. With no stimulus to breathe, respirations cease. This is usually seen in comatose patients and overall is rare. Never withhold oxygen for fear of causing respiratory arrest in a COPD patient with acute hypoxia. Simply watch for subsequent arrest and be aware that it can happen. A hypoxic patient needs to be given oxygen. Although rare, it does demonstrate hypoxic drive at its finest. It can ruin your whole afternoon.

So chronically pCO_2 climbs, giving a chronic respiratory acidosis on the pulmonary side of the equation. On the metabolic side, the kidneys will chronically retain bicarbonate to "counter" the respiratory acidosis with a metabolic alkalosis. This "compensation" serves well for years and very high pCO_2 readings can be seen (in conjunction with high bicarbonate readings) in an outwardly fairly healthy-appearing chronic lung patient.

It is a critical point in a COPD patient's course of illness, however, when the pCO_2 begins to climb. This is called hypercarbia (also known as hypercapnia). A normal pO_2 is greater than 80. A normal pCO_2 is 40 (range 35 to 45). When the patient "joins the 50-50 club," the pCO_2 has climbed above 50 and the pO_2 has dropped below 50. A chronic lung patient who is hypoxic and cannot sufficiently blow down their pCO_2 with maximum respiratory effort (hyperventilation) is in big trouble. If acute, a "50-50" patient frequently is ready for intubation and respirator support. Watch these "oncology patients in training" carefully—they are unpredictable.

D. Reactive Airway Disease (RADz)

RADZ, also known as **asthma,** is a common ailment. There are two major components to the pathophysiology of asthma: the **bronchoconstriction** caused by hyper-reactivity of the smooth muscle in the walls of the bronchioles, and the **inflammatory changes** in the respiratory mucosa leading to thick mucous plugging. Both cause air trapping. There is severe restriction of the outflow of air from the lungs. One classically hears diffuse multi-tonal musical wheezing on auscultation of the lungs (assuming that enough air is moving in and out of the lungs to make any noise at all).

Remember that CO_2 diffuses more readily than O_2. Asthma patients frequently hyperventilate during an acute attack. With oxygen supplementation hypoxia is not usually a problem. When present the patient is commonly near death. More subtle and "sneaky" is the pCO_2.

When you see a patient in acute asthmatic exacerbation, breathing at a rate of say 40 respirations per minute, be VERY WARY of a "normal pCO_2." At a respiratory rate of 40, a person should blow the pCO_2 down to well below normal. A "normal" pCO_2 in this setting is relatively HIGH. DO NOT be fooled by a "normal" reading. Such a patient may be imminently ready to crash. Be ready with respiratory support and assisted ventilation.

E. DKA

In diabetic ketoacidosis a patient generally has long-standing type I diabetes. Insufficient insulin is present to move glucose into the cells. The glucose in the vascular compartment therefore climbs. Meanwhile, the cells turn to burning fat in a relatively anaerobic process. High ketones and acidosis (metabolic acidosis) ensue.

Metabolic acids accumulate. A metabolic acidosis is seen as a low bicarbonate and a low pH. The respiratory system will try to compensate by "blowing off" CO_2. The patient will be hyperventilating and complaining of dyspnea and frequently of chest (or abdominal) discomfort.

A patient in DKA with no prior respiratory diagnosis will present as an acute metabolic acidosis with a compensating respiratory alkalosis (hyperventilation). There will be no hypoxia until well advanced.

Obviously, DKA presents more troubles than simple metabolic acidosis. All of the anomalies are big-time interrelated. There are five entities in DKA that all need to be addressed simultaneously in the acute management:

1. Hyperglycemia
2. Ketonemia with anaerobic metabolism
3. Metabolic acidosis
4. Hypokalemia and hyponatremia
5. Dehydration/hyperosmolarity/hypovolemia

Some other common states that can give metabolic acidosis and are therefore on the list for differential diagnosis are:

1. Lactic acidosis
2. Aspirin poisoning
3. Methanol ingestion (rare since Prohibition was repealed)
4. Paraldehyde overdose (I can't remember the last time I've seen this junk used)
5. Ethylene glycol poisoning (sucking antifreeze)
6. Renal failure/kidney disease
7. Protracted diarrhea

8. Ileostomy, colostomy, and some bowel diseases
9. Starvation ketosis
10. Alcoholic ketosis (whoops)

F. Code Arrest

In cardiopulmonary arrest, a two-sided problem emerges. The heart stops supplying an adequate flow and pressure. This leads to tissue hypoperfusion and a subsequent shift to anaerobic metabolism. Lactic and other acids climb giving an overall metabolic acidosis.

Secondly, the lungs stop their performance. Carbon dioxide is no longer adequately eliminated and accumulates. ("CO_2 is an acid.") This leads to a respiratory acidosis.

So, one sees a "combined" metabolic and respiratory acidosis in the acute code arrest patient. Because it is combined, there can be no compensation or correction attempts by the major systems. The acidosis is typically very ugly.

Cardiopulmonary resuscitation (CPR) with chest compressions and assisted ventilations can only improve the circulatory and ventilatory status. They don't fix it.

In years gone by, sodium bicarbonate was given in abundance during a code. This attacked the acidosis from the metabolic side of the equation. In recovery, the renal function is frequently compromised and these patients often could not get rid of all the bicarbonate. Prolonged coma, brain edema, seizures, paralysis and other problems were common. More modernly the respiratory side of the acidosis is targeted to treat the acidemia during a code. A code patient now is hyperventilated to drive pCO_2 down and hold the acidosis in check. Bicarbonate is given more judiciously. If the patient is on a ventilator in the recovery phase, the pH can be normalized with little effort by adjusting respiratory settings for rate and tidal volumes.

In a code keep in mind there will likely be a severe combined acidosis with little chance of endogenous compensation. The acidemic heart is very prone to dysrhythmias and will not defibrillate well. Concentrate efforts to normalize pH by securing the airway early, oxygenating fully, and consider hyperventilating the patient. Hopefully, you will have many patients survive into the recovery phase.

IV

METHOD OF MADNESS

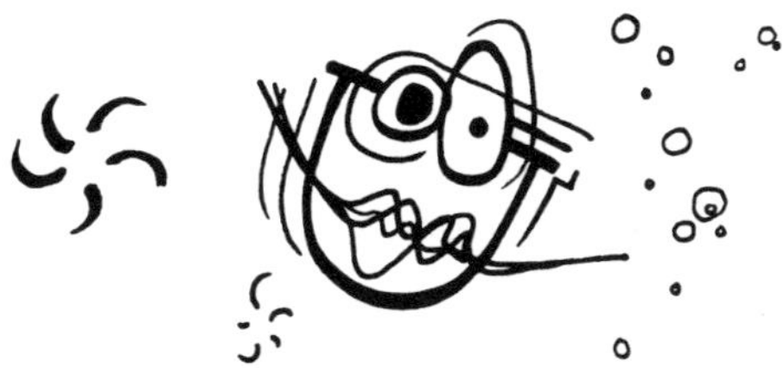

The following is a systematic method of reading ABG's. There is an order to the technique. Follow through each step in the same sequence on each set of blood gas results you interpret. Have the numbers read to you in this order when ABG results are called per telephone. Soon you'll have the proper interpretation before you can hang up the phone.

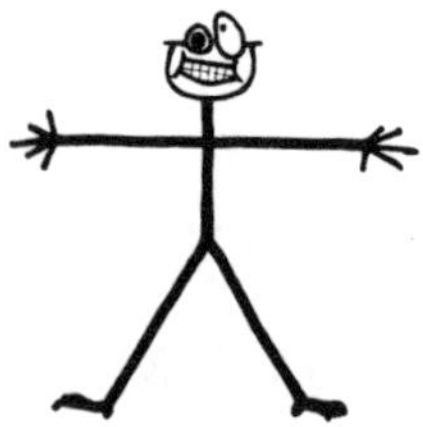

Meet Fred. Note that he is anatomically correct (anencephalic male). You should draw Fred before getting ABG numbers.

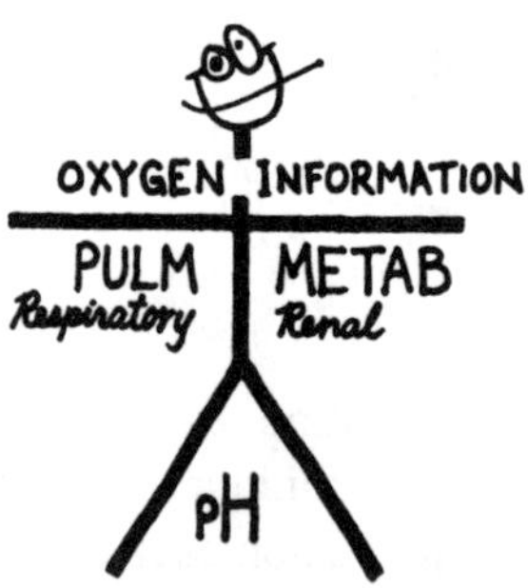

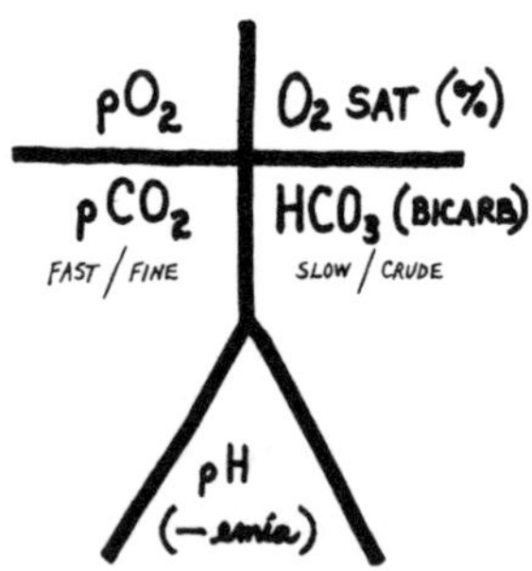

Place oxygen information on Fred's shoulders. Put the pO_2 on his right shoulder and O_2 SATURATION on his left. The overall acid-base balance goes between his legs. This is pH. Put the respiratory component (pCO_2) in his right armpit and put the metabolic/renal component (bicarb) in the left armpit. Bicarbonate is written HCO_3.

The **pO_2** is the pressure exerted by the oxygen gas in arterial blood. It is a very accurate indicator of lung function. Use pO_2 to call or rule out hypoxia. An acceptable value is 80 or greater. A normal pO_2 is around 95 at twenty years of age. However, over the age of twenty, a person normally drops the pO_2 by 3 every ten years. The formula would therefore be:

$$\text{NORMAL } pO_2 = 95 - \left[\frac{\text{AGE} - 20}{10}(\times 3)\right]$$

The **O_2SAT** is the percent of Hgb that is saturated with oxygen. This too tells a great deal about lung performance. In hypoxia the number is more sensitive than pO_2. A very small change in O_2 SAT may lead to a big change in pO_2, especially as the O_2 SAT falls below 90%. You should watch both and become familiar with how they relate to each other through experience. Once seasoned, you can monitor either one.

pH is a logarithmic value reflecting the overall acid-base balance. The normal pH in arterial blood is 7.40 with a normal range of 7.35 to 7.45. Look to pH to tell acidemia or alkalemia. Remember the suffix -emia means, "in the blood overall." Do not confuse it with acidosis or alkalosis. The suffix -osis signifies a diagnosis.

The respiratory information in the right armpit is the **pCO_2**. It is an acid. It diminishes as breathing accelerates and accumulates as respirations fail. The normal values and ranges are strikingly similar to the pH. Normal is 40 with a normal range of 35-45. Remember that the pulmonary side of the equation is the fast fine tuning.

Bicarbonate or **HCO_3** is the metabolic information for acid base balance. Recall that it is the slow crude control. You will see that the bicarbonate value on the ABG report can actually change fairly quickly. Bicarbonate already in the body can be available and upon short notice accept acid ions. This available HCO_3 then gets "used up" in the buffering process. Be aware that true changes in TOTAL body bicarbonate take time and adequate kidney function. Bicarbonate range that's normal is the perfect dating age for your children: 22 to 26 with an average of 24.

Base excess (or **BE**) tells the available base at the time of the draw. A negative number indicates a "negative excess" (i.e., a deficit). I don't pay much attention to BE. It hasn't very often helped tell me more about the patient. Put the BE (if you want to) on Fred's left knee. You can write the O_2 being given to the patient at the time of draw on his right knee.

Read ABG's in the following order. First draw Fred. Then write the values in their proper position as

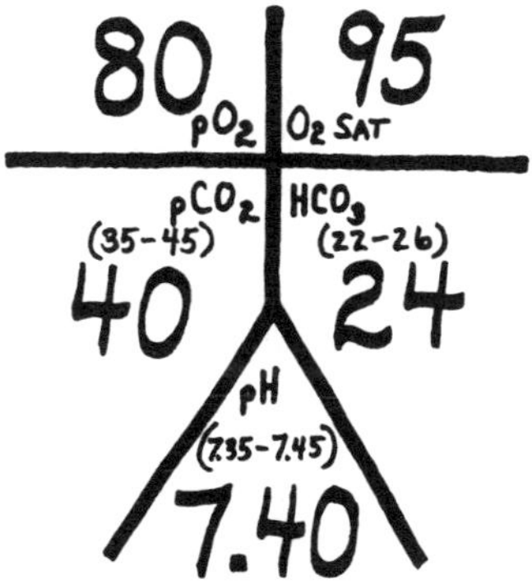

described above. Begin with pO_2 and then O_2 SAT to decide the quality of oxygenation. If poor, this needs to be of paramount concern. If oxygen isn't getting into arterial blood on its way to the brain and body, then nothing else matters. A low oxygenation during a code has alerted me to the fact that the ET tube had drifted into the right mainstem bronchus. Evaluate oxygenation first. Note the status as "normal" or "nasty" and WRITE IT to the side of Fred. Move on.

Jump down between Fred's legs to see the pH. Note whether there is "normal pH," "acidemia," or "alkalemia." Write this to the side of Fred as well. The next two steps will be for the purpose of explaining the pH. Once you identify the overall acid-base balance with pH, you will go on to the pCO_2 to find out what part the respiratory component is playing. Knowing that, you will then proceed to the bicarbonate to explain

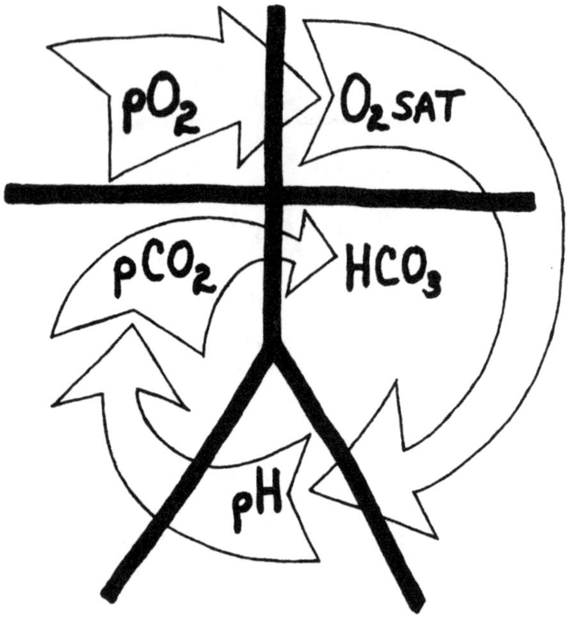

the metabolic system's role in making the pH what it currently is.

So, we next go to Fred's right armpit. If the pCO_2 is normal, the respiratory system is not contributing in any way to any abnormality seen in pH. Any change would be purely metabolic. If the pCO_2 is low, there is a RESPIRATORY ALKALOSIS. Write "R. ALK." under the oxygen notation and pH notation to the side of Fred. If the pCO_2 is high, there is a RESPIRATORY ACIDOSIS. Write "R. ACID." under the oxygen and pH notation to the side of Fred. If normal write "R. NORMAL." It is very important to note that there can be a respiratory alkalosis REGARDLESS of whether the pH is normal, high, or low. Likewise there can be a respiratory acidosis regardless of whether there is normal pH, alkalemia, or acidemia. A respiratory alkalosis proves hyperventilation. A respiratory acidosis proves hypoventilation. You now know what part the respiratory system is playing in the overall pH change (if any).

Now check Fred's left armpit to evaluate the metabolic (renal) component. If the bicarbonate (HCO_3) is low, there is a METABOLIC ACIDOSIS. Write "M. ACID" to the side of Fred under the respiratory information. If the bicarbonate is high, there is a METABOLIC ALKALOSIS present. Write "M. ALK" to the side of Fred.

The pH should now be fully explained by both the respiratory and metabolic systems. Let's do some examples.

Wait. When I hit this stuff too hard all at once, everything gets crooked in my head. Take five and come back with some scratch paper.

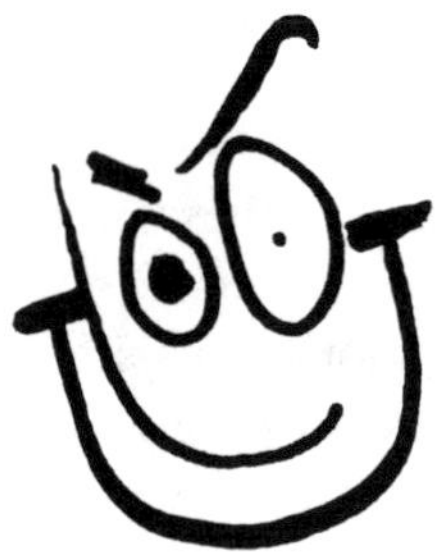

4a. EXAMPLE:

Let's go. Draw Fred. Write the values for this first sample in their proper position. The pO_2 is 88 and O_2 SATURATION is 97%. The pH is 7.39. The pCO_2 is 40 and HCO_3 is 25.

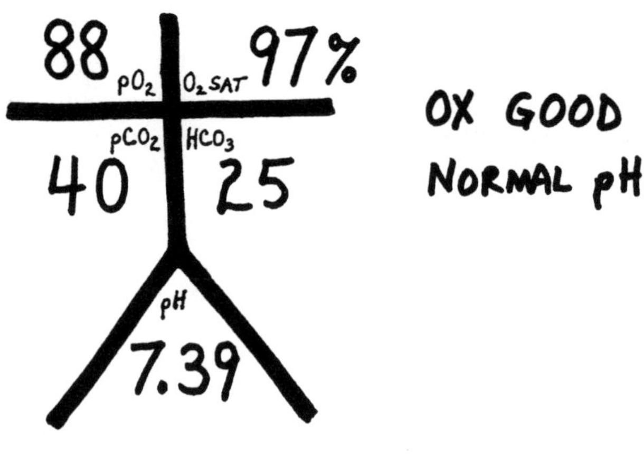

Begin with the pO_2. It is higher than normal and therefore fine. The O_2 SATURATION is likewise normal or better. At this point write "OX GOOD" or some other such phrase to indicate the oxygenation meets (or surpasses) muster. Next check the pH and note that it is normal. Write "NORMAL pH" under the oxygenation notation. Move to the pCO_2 and see that there is no alteration in the respiratory component. The metabolic is then checked and we see that HCO_3 is normal as well. This is a normal ABG.

4b. EXAMPLE:

The next example is a thirty-seven-year-old female complaining of dyspnea. The following are the ABG values. The bicarb is 23. The pO_2 is 104. The pH is 7.53 and the pCO_2 is 24. The O_2 SATURATION is 99%.

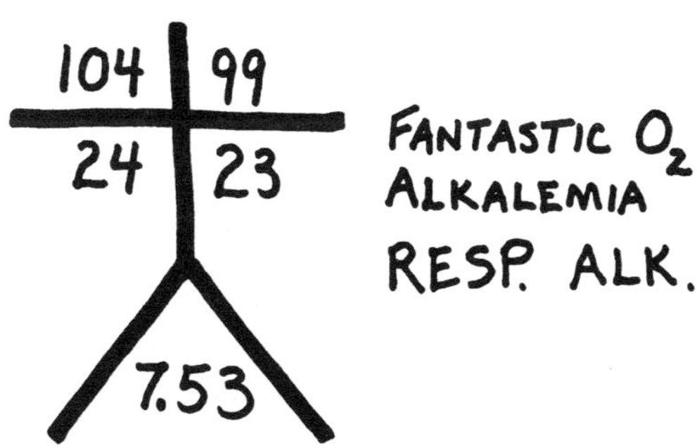

Begin, as always, with the pO_2. It is great and so is the O_2 SAT. Write "FANTASTIC O_2" to the side of Fred. Next check the pH. The pH is high, indicating an alkalemia. Write "ALKALEMIA" (NOT alkalosis) below the oxygenation note to the side of Fred. Now look to the pCO_2 to determine how the respiratory component is contributing to the pH change. The pCO_2 is very low at 24, down from a normal of 40. The pCO_2 is therefore "blown down" and this defines hyperventilation. A respiratory alkalosis is therefore present. Write "R. ALK" below the "ALKALEMIA." Next go to the bicarb, which is normal. Therefore, the metabolic system is contributing nothing and all abnormalities in pH are due to the respiratory system's contribution. This goes nicely with the respiratory alkalosis explaining the overall alkalemia present. This is a classic patient with acute hyperventilation syndrome and no underlying cardiopulmonary disease. This is a "pure" respiratory alkalosis in that the metabolic system has not had time to "compensate" by losing HCO_3. The metabolic component added nothing to the pH change.

4c. EXAMPLE:

In this next example, we have a patient with an acute heart attack. The patient has longstanding COPD and CHF as well as a current pneumonia prior to the myocardial infarction. The patient suffered cardiopulmonary arrest and CPR is in progress. Oxygen is being administered through an ET tube at full flow 100%. Draw Fred and fill in these values.

The pH is 7.17. The pO_2 is only 50. The bicarbonate is 16 and the O_2 SATURATION is 62. The pCO_2 is 52. Base Excess is -9.

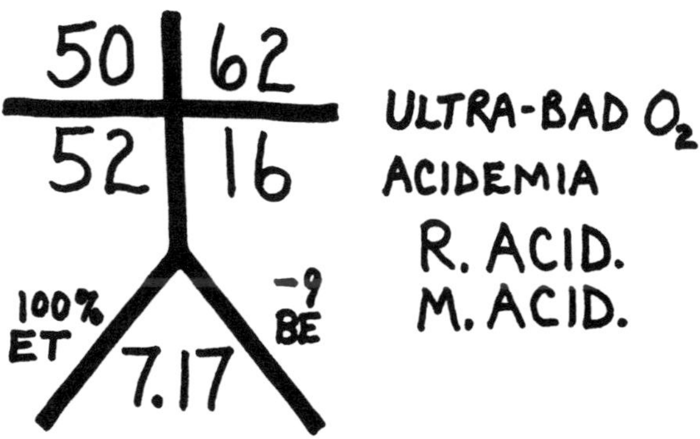

Begin with the oxygenation information. Write the administered oxygen on the right knee. This is a lot of O_2. The pO_2 is very low for such a high administered O_2. (50 pO_2 is even low for a normal person breathing room air.) Write "ULTRA-BAD O_2" to the side of Fred.

Per protocol next look at the pH. Note that there is

significant acidemia and write "ACIDEMIA" below the oxygenation. Now go to the pulmonary component. The pCO_2 is high indicating hypoventilation. The lungs aren't functioning well since there is hypoxia and CO_2 retention. This is respiratory acidosis with the high pCO_2. Write "R. ACID." below the "ACIDEMIA" notation. Next check the metabolic component by noting the bicarbonate. The HCO_3 is low, showing a metabolic acidosis (low metabolic base means metabolic acidosis). Write "M. ACID." below the respiratory notation. Therefore this example shows an overall acidemia of both the respiratory and metabolic systems. This is a "combined" respiratory and metabolic acidosis with hypoxia. Note the patient is in the "50-50 club" and in big trouble.

4d. EXAMPLE:

This next set is from a sixty-eight-year-old female with an extensive smoking history. She feels great and gets ABG's during pre-operative medical clearance for elective foot surgery.

The Base Excess (BE) is +6.2. The pO_2 on room air (RA) is 67. Bicarb is 32. The pCO_2 is high at 52 and the O_2 SAT is 88%. The pH is 7.39.

This is an interesting one. It's also a common sight. Remember that the patient is in no acute distress. These numbers are therefore likely to be usual for her.

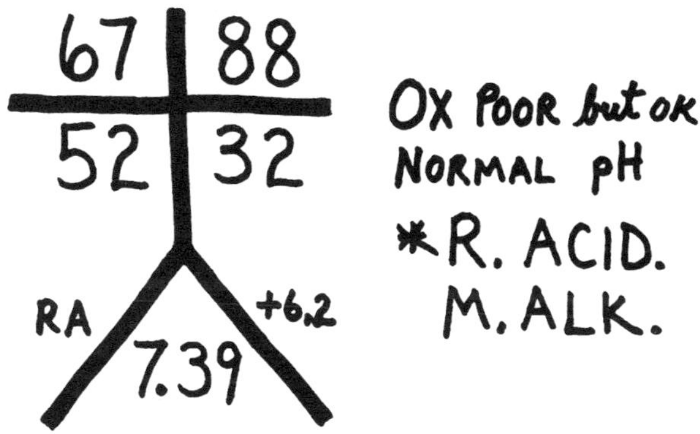

Begin with the oxygenation data. The pO_2 is low, but over 50. There is a corresponding low O_2 SAT. This oxygenation status is poor but acutely "ok" in this long-time smoker.

Moving to the pH, we see it's damned near normal! There is no acidemia nor alkalemia. Write "NORMAL pH" off to the side. (I sure hope you are writing the notes to the side. It will be important later.) Next check the respiratory system's contribution. There is a high pCO_2. CO_2 is an acid. There is a respiratory acidosis present. (Write "R ACID.")

Let's pause. Without even looking at the metabolic contribution, it's already clear that the metabolic system *must* be giving an alkalosis. That would be necessary to offset the respiratory acidosis that we already know about to explain the normal pH.

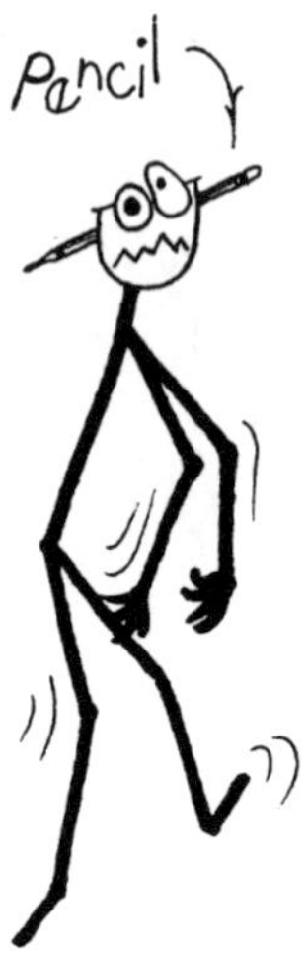

Looking at the HCO_3 we confirm that it is high at 32, showing an excess of base, i.e., a metabolic alkalosis.

Remember that if only one system is affected and the other is normal, the condition is termed "pure," i.e., pure respiratory alkalosis in which the metabolic is normal. When both systems are giving the same type of pH shift, we call it "combined," i.e., combined respiratory and metabolic acidosis. Lastly, when both systems are involved but opposite in their pH shifts, it is said to be a "compensating" state.

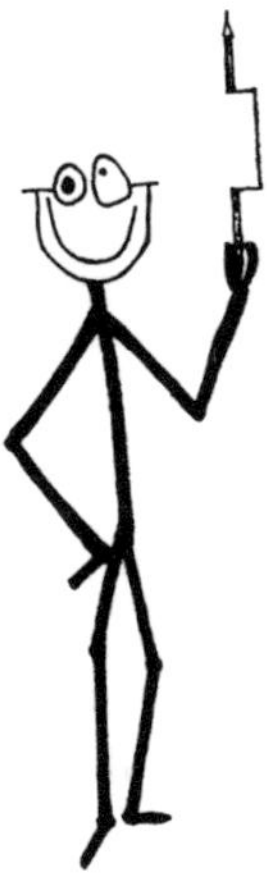

But therein lies the rub. Which came first, the chicken or the egg? Which is compensating which? Is the acidosis trying to correct the alkalosis or is the alkalosis attempting to fix the acidosis? Three rules should be employed to decide which is compensating in these cases:

Rule #1: CHECK THE HISTORY. Many times, as in

this example, the answer is in the history. This patient has chronic lung disease. The chronic hypercarbia defines chronic respiratory acidosis. With all the CO_2 retention and acidemia, the renal system begins holding onto bicarbonate to counter it with a chronic metabolic alkalosis. Therefore, the R. ACID is the primary problem and the M. ALK is compensating. (I like to put an asterisk beside the primary problem.)

Rule #2. WATCH YOUR SPEED. The difference in time that it takes the two systems to respond can frequently give you a clue as to the primary pathology. Assuming you already have a diagnosis, simply remember that the respiratory system can compensate quickly, but it takes the renal system much longer to compensate. In the present example, you can conclude that the respiratory failure is chronic since the renal system had time to accumulate bicarb to compensate.

Rule #3: A FIX IS RARELY COMPLETE. Whenever a primary problem is compensated endogenously (by the patient themselves), the result is rarely complete and virtually never over-corrected. In this case the respiratory acidosis was chronic and the primary problem. The metabolic alkalosis was compensating. Note the pH was 39—ever so slightly in the acidemic direction, helping to confirm that the acidosis (respiratory acidosis in this case) was the primary problem.

4e. EXAMPLE:

A sixty-eight-year-old female with no cardiopulmonary diagnosis has chronic renal failure. She comes in ill and dehydrated. The O_2 SATURATION is 93%. Bicarb is 11 and pO_2 82. The pCO_2 is 40 with a pH of 7.25. Work the problem, then check your answer.

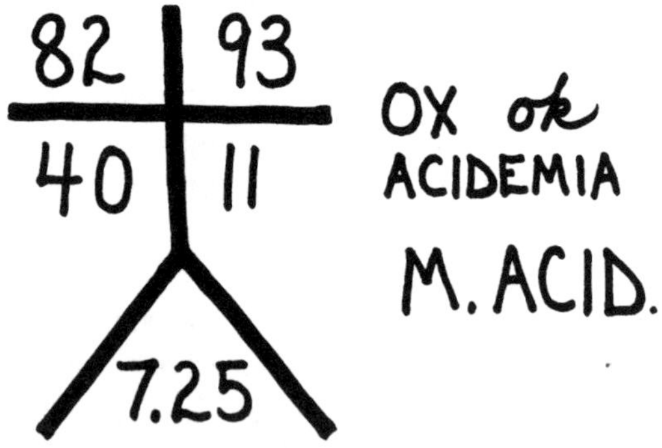

With the pCO_2 normal, all the alteration in pH must be due to the metabolic system. Sure enough, the HCO_3 is low at eleven. This is a pure metabolic acidosis due to renal failure.

This concludes the basic technique of reading ABG's. Always follow the sequence. Write the notes to the side. The next chapter will add a new layer of preciseness to this very same method. If you're not interested in learning the math and simply want to use the "on-sight" method already presented, then fine! Ignore the teaching in the next chapter. HOWEVER, THERE ARE EXAMPLES IN THE NEXT CHAPTER THAT ARE QUITE VALUABLE. (To keep this here book short, I stuck only half the examples into each chapter. The examples in the next chapter were never meant to be passed over.) If you elect not to learn the mathematical correlation, be sure to apply the on-sight method to the examples in chapter V. The answers will be provided.

V

BY THE NUMBERS

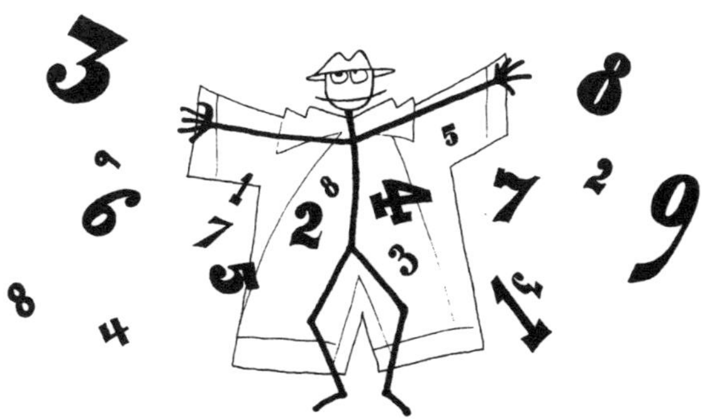

A more exact determination of ABG results can be accomplished by acknowledging a single rule: "For every change of 10 in pCO_2, the pH will change by .08 in the opposite direction." Memorize this phrase.

Stated as a formula:

$$\frac{\overset{\text{OPPOSITE}}{\Delta pCO_2(.08)}}{10} = \overset{\text{OPPOSITE}}{\Delta}\ pH$$

We already knew that as the pCO_2 goes up, the pH goes down and vice versa. ("CO_2 is an ACID.") This rule simply tells you by how much.

There's only one way to teach this stuff. Let's do it.

5a. EXAMPLE:

A sixty-year-old woman with no history of heart or lung disease suddenly presents with an acute myocardial infarction. It is early in the code arrest that soon followed. The ABG's show a bicarb of 26. The O_2 SAT is 41%. The pH is 7.20 and there is a pO_2 of 25. The pCO_2 is up to 65. Write it.

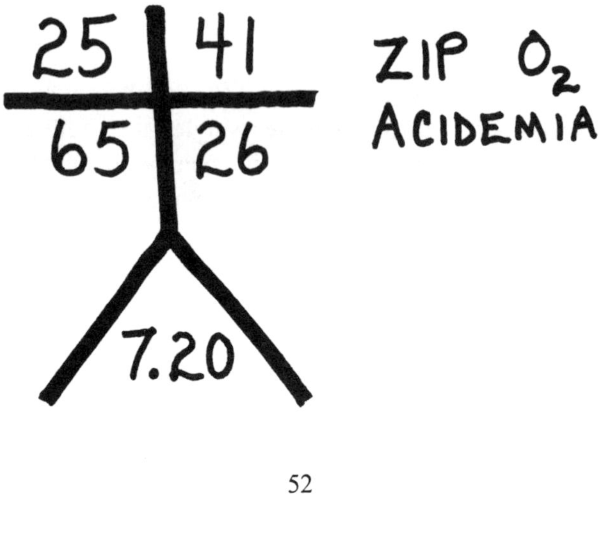

Looking at the pO_2 and then the O_2 SAT, one sees poor oxygenation. Write "ZIP O_2," to the right of Fred. Next we see the pH is 7.20. Low pH is acidemia. Write "ACIDEMIA." The pH is lower than normal by .2, so draw an arrow downward below pH and write .2 beside it. This notation "↓.2" means that the pH is "down below normal by .2." It does NOT mean that the pH value is or should be .2. (Although in this case by chance it happens to be.)

As per usual, look next at the pCO_2. It is 65 defining hypoventilation and establishing respiratory acidosis. Write "R. ACID." The pCO_2 is "up above normal by 25" so draw an upwards arrow and "25" next to the pCO_2.

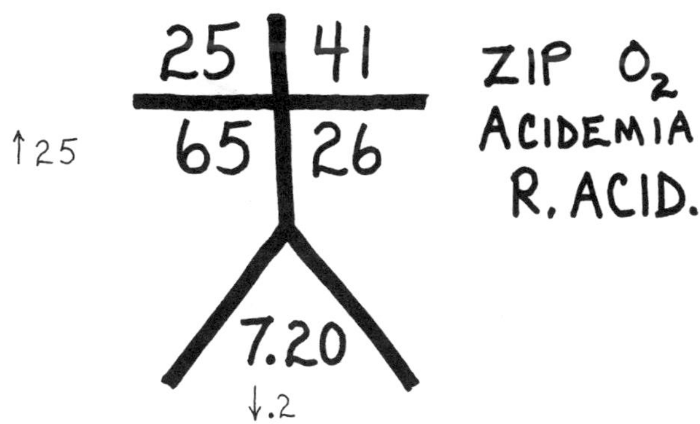

This notation, "↑25" means the pCO_2 is 25 higher than normal. It does NOT mean the pCO_2 value is or should be 25. (Nothing will screw ya up faster'n twistin' this around.)

Now the rule comes into play. Recite it as you write the following: "For every change of 10 in pCO_2. . . . "

Divide the CHANGE in pCO_2 by 10 by moving the decimal point to the left one space. "For every change of 10 in pCO_2. . . . The pH will change by .08. . . . "

Multiply the 2.5 by .08 and arrive at .200. **This is the pH change expected given the pCO_2 change of 25.**

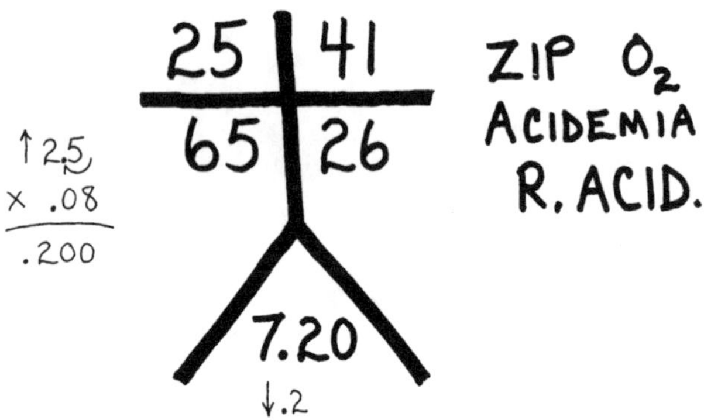

"For every change of 10 in pCO_2 the pH will change by .08 in the opposite direction." The pCO_2 is an acid and pH shows acidic change by lowering. Therefore the pH and pCO_2 will always move opposite each other. You wrote an arrow upwards to signify the increase in pCO_2. Therefore, make the change in pH of .200 with a downward arrow.

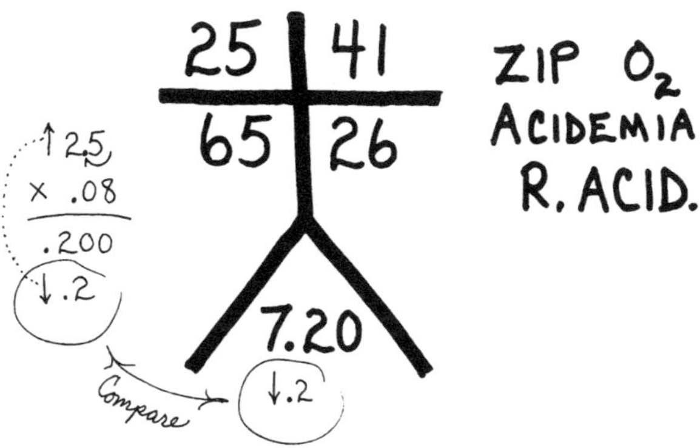

The notation " ↓.2" means that given the increase of 25 in pCO_2 the pH is expected to drop by .2. I like to circle this final value. Now compare it to the actual change in pH written earlier.

By our calculations the pCO_2 increase would be expected to drop the pH by .2. The pH is down by exactly .2. Therefore we conclude that ALL the change in pH (acidemia) can be attributed to the change in pCO_2. In other words, the respiratory system accounts for all the pH change. There is no metabolic component. The

“R. ACID” written earlier stands and is alone. This is a case of pure respiratory acidosis.

By the way . . . the ET tube was in the esophagus.

In summary, as you recite the rule, “For every change of ten in pCO_2 . . . the pH will change by .08 . . . in the opposite direction,” you will move the decimal one space left (divide by ten) in the pCO_2 change value, then multiply it by .08, then place an opposite arrow next to the result. This mathematical result tells you the expected change in pH given the pCO_2 reading. This result is compared to the actual change in pH. If it doesn’t compare closely, then any further change MUST BE due to alterations in the metabolic system.

Ain’t this more fun than being in a poker game with a planeload of Swedish dyslexics?

5b. EXAMPLE:

This next patient is a thirty-six-year-old male in a car accident. He was severely injured with chest trauma. During a brief code arrest, he was given 2 amps of sodium bicarb. He was intubated and is in the ICU on a respirator now. ABG’s are drawn.

The HCO_3 is 38 and pO_2 106. O_2 SAT is 100%. The pCO_2 is only 24 and pH 7.68.

The oxygenation is excellent. The pH shows an alkalemia and is up by .28. Mark “↑.28” below the pH.

The pCO_2 shows hyperventilation (respiratory alkalosis) and is down by 16. Mark "↓16" beside the pCO_2.

"For every change of 10 in pCO_2 . . . " (change the 16 to 1.6), " . . . The pH will change by .08 . . . " (multiply by .08 to reach .128—round to .13), " . . . in the opposite direction . . . " (place the upwards arrow because the pCO_2 change was downward).

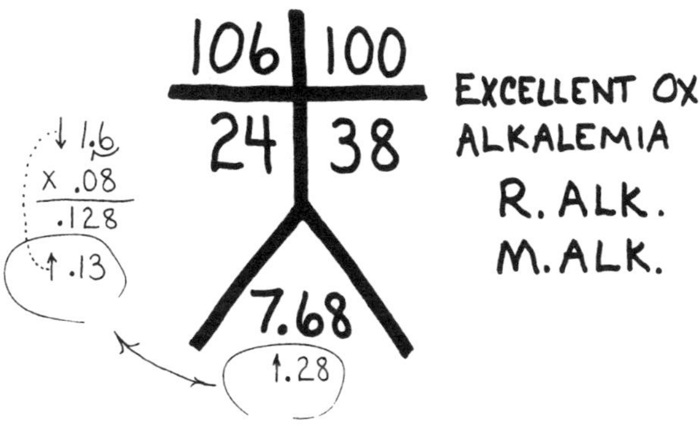

This patient had a drop of pCO_2 to 24. Given this, it is predicted that the pH should increase by .13. Comparing this prediction to the actual change in pH, we see that the pH is even higher than the predicted elevation. It is up by .28, with an increase of only .13 predicted by the respiratory component. That means an additional elevation of .15 is present. This is an additional alkalosis and it is attributed to the metabolic system. There is a metabolic alkalosis as well. (Write it under "R. ALK.")

This is therefore a combined respiratory and metabolic alkalosis. He was given a bit much bicarbonate during the code arrest and is now being hyperventilated on the respirator.

5c. EXAMPLE:

The next case is a fifty-two-year-old alcoholic male smoker with a history of bleeding ulcers. He's had severe dyspepsia for the last several weeks with occasional coffee-ground emesis. He comes to the hospital ill. The respiratory rate is 26. He is anemic.

ABG's show a pH of 7.62 with O_2 SAT of 88% and a pO_2 of 64. The bicarb is 40 as is the pCO_2.

Work through the problem and then check your answer.

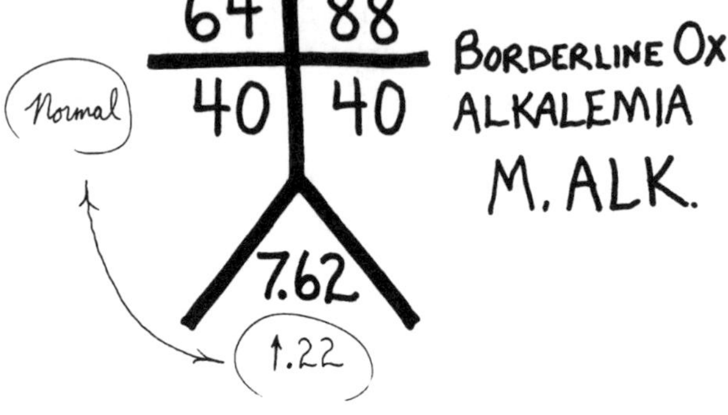

You should find a pure metabolic alkalosis. The pCO_2 is normal, so all the alteration in pH must be due to the metabolic system (all .22 increase of it).

Of further interest is that the pO_2 is notably low for an O_2 SAT of 88%. This is explained by the anemia. The red-cell mass is low, so even with 88% of the hemoglobin saturated, he can still only mount an O_2 partial pressure of 64. Additionally, there is a relative hypercarbia. Remember that the patient is tachypnic at 26 breaths per minute. At this rate, he should have been able to blow down the pCO_2. He did not. This is therefore a relative hypercarbia and good evidence of overall poor lung function from his smoking. Notice that you do NOT count relative hypercarbia in diagnosing acid-base anomalies. Use the information to make clinical decisions.

Did you conclude that the pure metabolic alkalosis was due to his ingestion of industrial-strength doses of absorbable antacid?

5d. EXAMPLE:

This case is of a previously healthy sixteen-year-old female who ingested an enormous quantity of aspirin. She is pale, diaphoretic, and complains of "not being able to feel my body." She is quite lethargic. Oxygen is being given by mask at 4 liters. Vitals are: BP 104/72, P 146, R 58, T 98.0° F.

The pCO_2 is 10. O_2 SAT is 92% with pH of 7.08. Base excess (BE) is −25.4. The pO_2 is 108. Bicarb is 4.

Run through it, then check your answer.

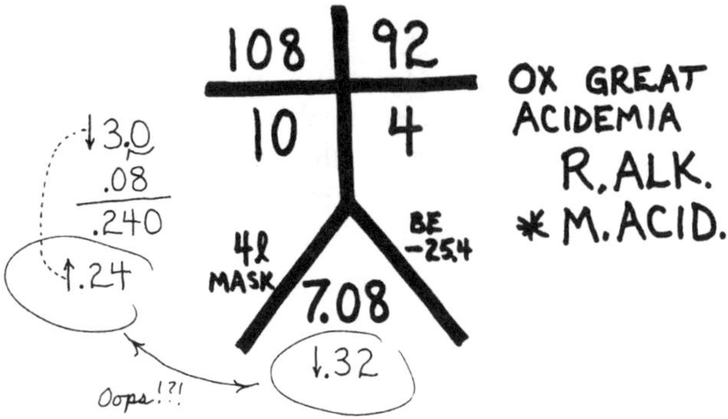

There is a profound acidemia. Since the metabolic and respiratory systems are shifted in opposite directions (acidic in one and basic in the other), there is a compensating state present.

The change in pCO_2 predicts a rise in pH of .24. In reality there is an actual *drop* in pH of .32. One concludes that there must be a kick-butt metabolic acidosis present. Another way to "identify" what the metabolic system is causing in this case would be to ask the question, "What if the respiratory system was normal and contributing nothing?" Imagine the pCO_2 normal at 40 and erase out the .24 elevation predicted in pH. The true pH change would then be a decrease of .56 and pH would therefore be 6.84! You can think of the hyperventilation as "holding up" the pH from being much lower than it already is. When we move on to the bicarb of 4 and a BE of -25.4 (remember a negative number for base "excess" is a base deficit), it becomes quite believable that a significant metabolic acidosis is present.

Since the patient is overall acidemic, it is concluded that the acidosis is the main problem. There is, therefore, a metabolic acidosis with a partially compensating respiratory alkalosis. This fits nicely with the history and physical exam. The patient ingested large amounts of aspirin (salacylic acid) and is tachypic at 58.

You have now been exposed to all nine basic combinations of acid-base balance. In the compensating states, either the metabolic or respiratory system can be primary. For example, in a metabolic acidosis with res-

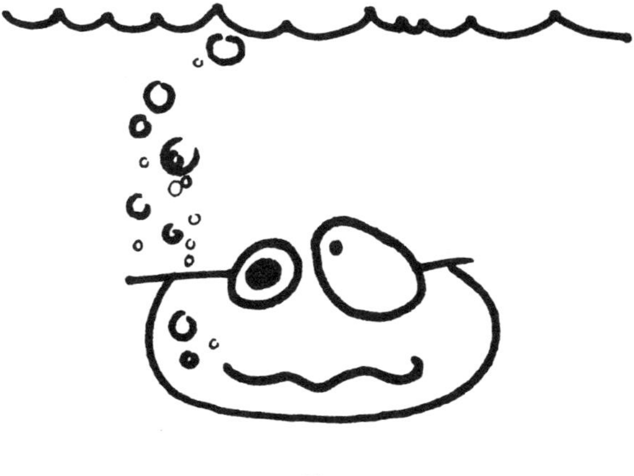

piratory alkalosis, there can be an overall acidemia or alkalemia (usually depending upon which is primary and which is compensating).

After a time, if you interpret ABG's often enough in your career, you'll be able to "do the math" in your head to arrive at accurate conclusions. Collect and analyze as many ABG results as you can. Always try to explain your results clinically. In compensating states determine which problem is primary and which is compensating.

Remember to take into account the three major components of the information found in an ABG result: 1) the oxygenation information, 2) the ability to rid the body of the waste gas CO_2, and 3) the acid-base balance. And never, NEVER! skydive naked during an electrical storm.

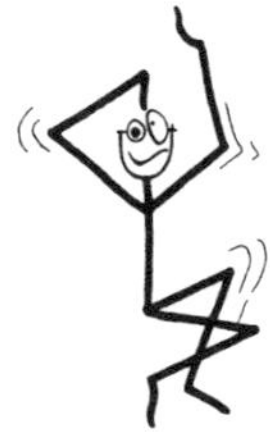

VI

PRACTICE MAKES PERFECT

You truly know something once you can teach it. Find the most intellectually challenged member of your healthcare study group and teach him ABG interpretation. Then you know it.

That last sample, by the way, was tough. Understand the compensating states and you're well on the way.

In this chapter we'll run through samples. Let's begin with putting the numbers to some of the examples in chapter IV. We'll skip examples that are all around normal, have normal pH, or normal pCO_2 (examples 4a, 4d, and 4e) since "doing the math" on such samples doesn't add much to

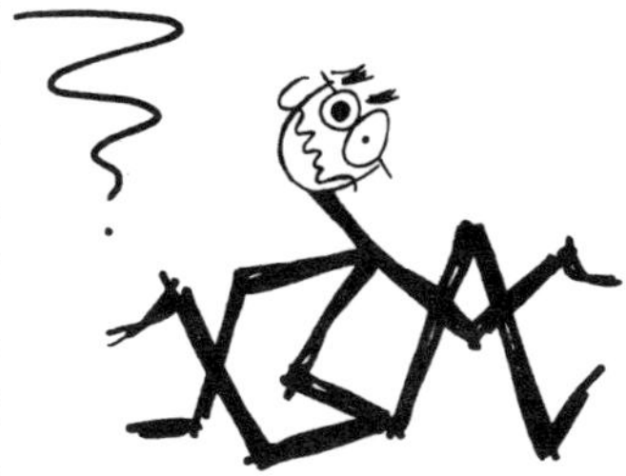

the interpretation. Do the figuring on the following, then check your answers.

4b. EXAMPLE: (from page 41)

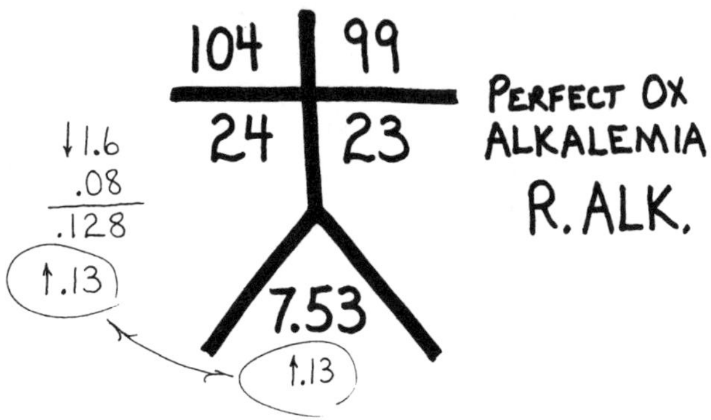

This is confirmed to be a pure respiratory alkalosis.

4c. EXAMPLE: (from page 42)

The respiratory acidosis accounts for a fall of .1 in pH. The remaining .13 fall in pH is due to the metabolic acidosis.

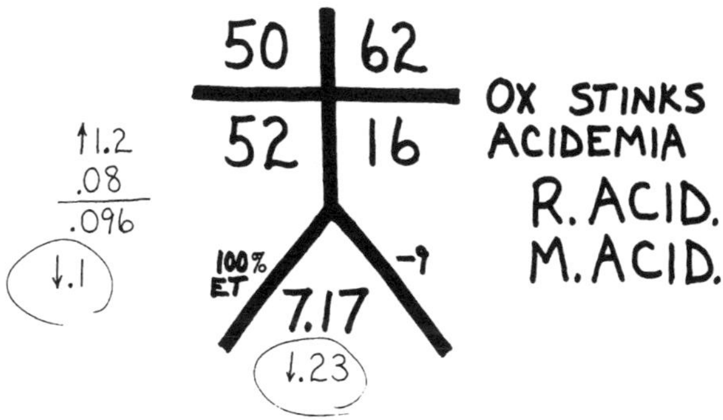

Now a pile of examples for your enjoyment.

6a. EXAMPLE:

A sixty-year-old man has COPD and a URI. Respiratory rate is 32 on 4 liters of O_2 by nasal cannula. BE is -2.5 with bicarb 19.0. The O_2 SAT is 98.3% and pO_2 100.4. The pCO_2 is 26. The pH is 7.47.

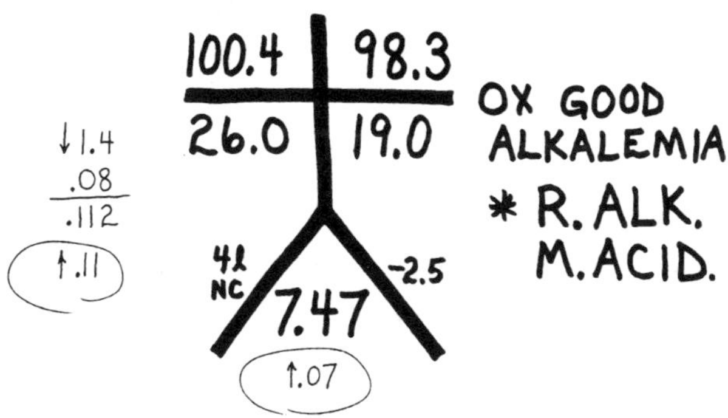

The change in pCO_2 predicts a pH elevation of .11. Actual pH elevated only .07—short by .04. The pH was lower by .04 due to a slight compensating metabolic acidosis. This patient's COPD has not been severe enough to cause chronic hypercarbia and subsequent chronic bicarb retention.

6b. EXAMPLE:

A code is in progress. There is a difficult arterial stick. The HCO_3 is 36 and pH 7.37. The O_2 SAT is 80%. The pCO_2 is 66 and pO_2 40. Can you be sure this is an arterial draw?

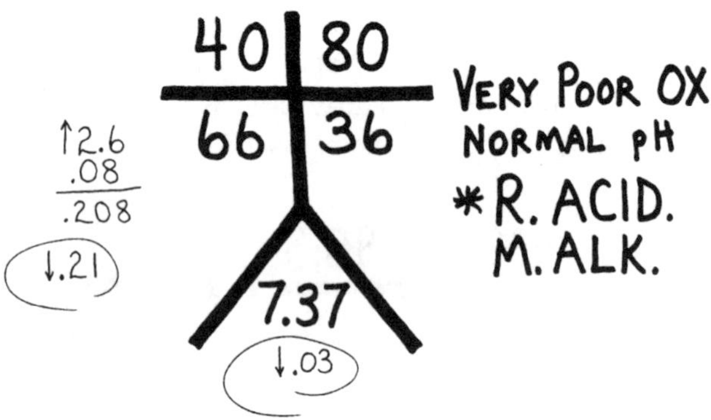

You can be sure this is in fact an arterial draw since the O_2 SAT is greater than 75. (See venous draw under PITFALLS in chapter I.) Long-standing lung trouble has probably led to chronic bicarbonate retention. The respiratory acidosis is primary, with a compensating metabolic alkalosis. Note how the actual pH drop is far less than predicted by the pCO_2 change and how the metabolic alkalosis "holds the pH up."

6c. EXAMPLE:

An anxious twenty-year-old female presents with dyspnea, pallor, and numb cheeks. She is tremulous as she arrives by ambulance. O_2 is being given by mask at 6 liters per minute.

ABG's are drawn in the ER and show a pO_2 of 128 and O_2 SAT of 99%. The pCO_2 is 26 and bicarb 22. The pH is 7.51.

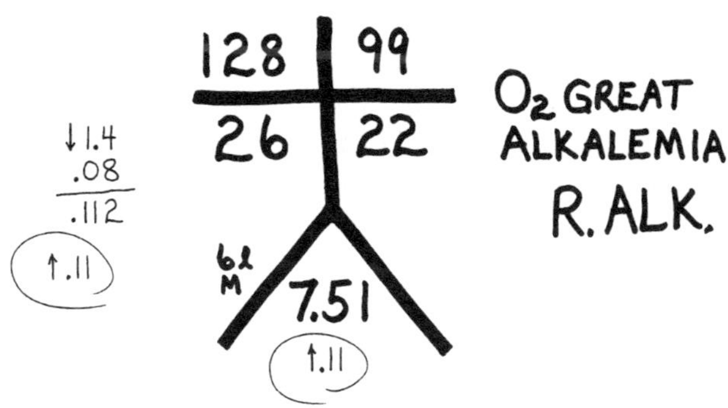

There is a pure respiratory alkalosis. This is hyperventilation syndrome.

6d. EXAMPLE:

A seventy-two-year-old female is dying of CHF. The ABG's show a pH of 7.09. Bicarb is 19.1 and pCO_2 is 62.8. The pO_2 is 65.1 and O_2 SAT 82.5%.

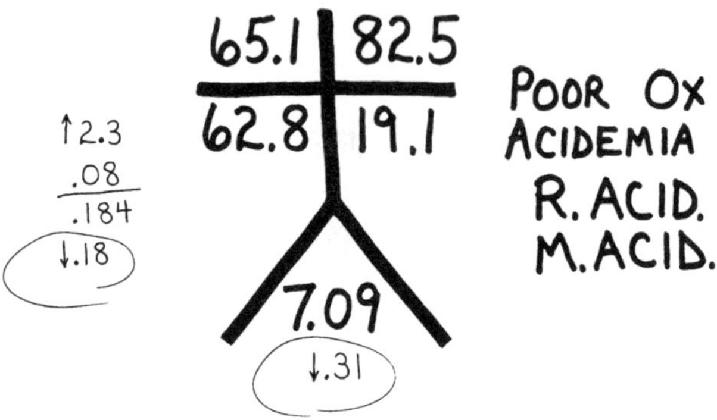

There is a combined metabolic and respiratory acidosis. The change in pCO_2 predicts a pH drop of .18. The actual drop is much more than that showing the additional metabolic component to the combined acidemia.

6e. EXAMPLE:

A forty-seven-year-old male arrives from an outside hospital with an unknown illness. He is comatose.

The pH is 7.26. The partial pressure of O_2 is 87 with an O_2 SAT of 96. HCO_3 is 13 and pCO_2 32.

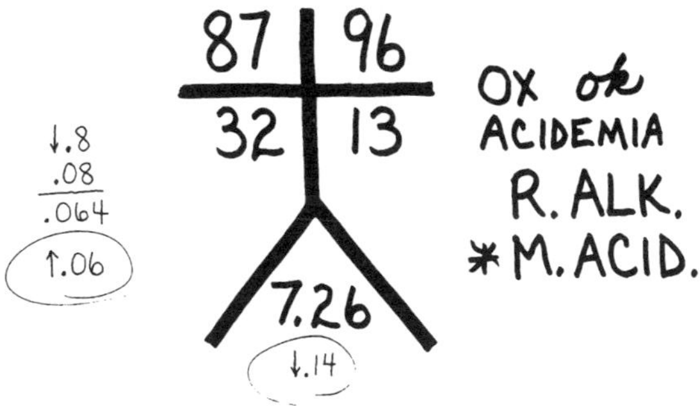

Acidemia is present. The respiratory system shows an alkalemia (hyperventilation) and predicts a *rise* in pH of .06. There is no actual rise in pH—rather a fall of .14. The metabolic system shows a pH fall of .20 (erase out the respiratory rise). The metabolic acidosis is primary with a compensatory respiratory alkalosis. The patient had a polysubstance ingestion.

6f. EXAMPLE:

A thirty-four-year-old male fireman is overcome by hot metallic fumes. He presents with chest pain and dyspnea. He is on 10 liters of O_2 by nasal cannula.

ABG's are drawn and show a pH of 7.56. The bicarb is 24.3 with a BE of -0.2. The pO_2 is 104.7 and O_2 SAT is 98.9. The pCO_2 is 21.4.

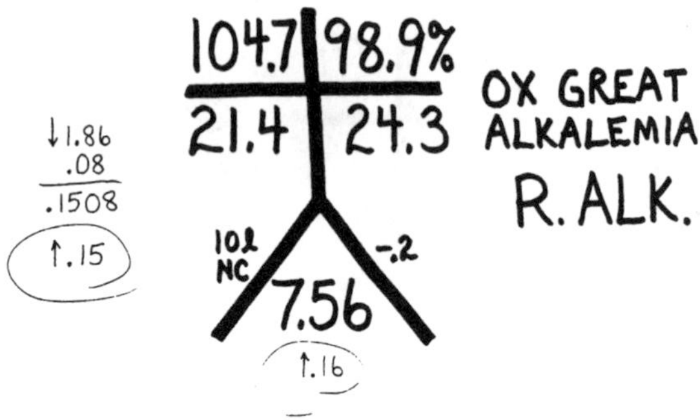

The expected change in pH closely matched the actual change. We called a simple pure respiratory alkalosis. He was admitted to the hospital for observation. Six hours later the patient crashed. Subsequent ABG's are shown in the next example.

6g. EXAMPLE:

The next ABG's were taken with the patient in worsening pulmonary edema. Respirations were 30.

The pH was 7.26. The pO_2 was 61 with an O_2 SAT of 88%. Bicarb shifted to 19 and pCO_2 climbed to 50.

There is now a combined metabolic and respiratory acidosis. The bicarb is being "used up" by the respiratory system's failing status. A hypoxia is now present. Sudden pulmonary edema is a lethal complication of acute inhalation injury. Never trust a fireman sucking hot black air.

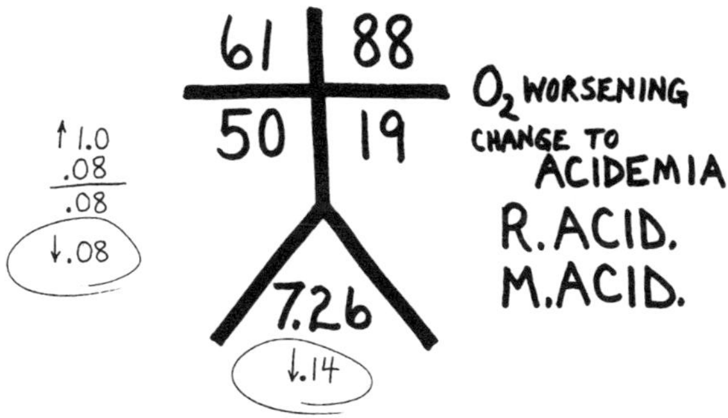

6h. EXAMPLE:

A thirty-one-year-old male presents with chest pain. O_2 is being delivered at 4 liters. He is severely dehydrated with a blood glucose of 822 and positive serum ketones.

The ABG's show a pH of 7.21 with bicarb of 4.9 and pCO_2 of 12.8. The pO_2 is 116.1 and O_2 SAT is 99.1.

This is DKA. The pCO_2 change predicts for the respiratory system a pH increase of .22. The actual pH change is a drop well into the acidemic range. The drop in pH due to the metabolic systems is therefore .41. This "hidden" acidemia is of course due to the metabolic system. This is a primary metabolic acidosis (diabetic ketoacidosis) with a valiant effort at compensation by the respiratory system.

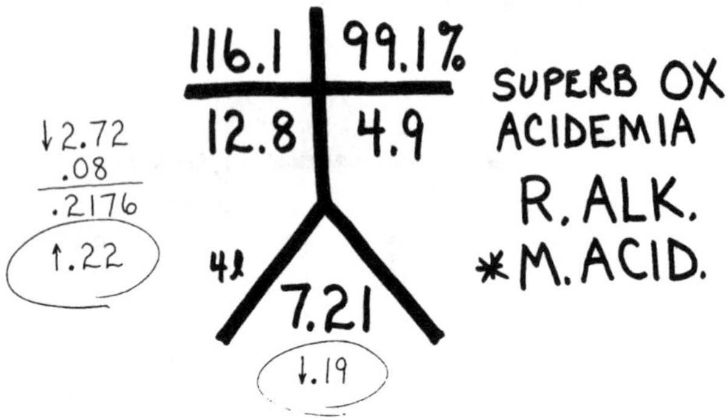

6i. EXAMPLE:

A healthy fifty-five-year-old woman with no ongoing diagnoses presents with shortness of breath. She just finished a three-day car trip. She's on no medicines, but has "arthritis pain" in her legs. The left calf is warm and tender. Respirations are 38.

ABG's show a pH of 7.60. The pO_2 is 64 and O_2 SAT 89%. The HCO_3 is 23. The pCO_2 is 16. She's on room air.

This is a pure respiratory alkalosis with hypoxia. She had a DVT of the calf and a small pulmonary embolus.

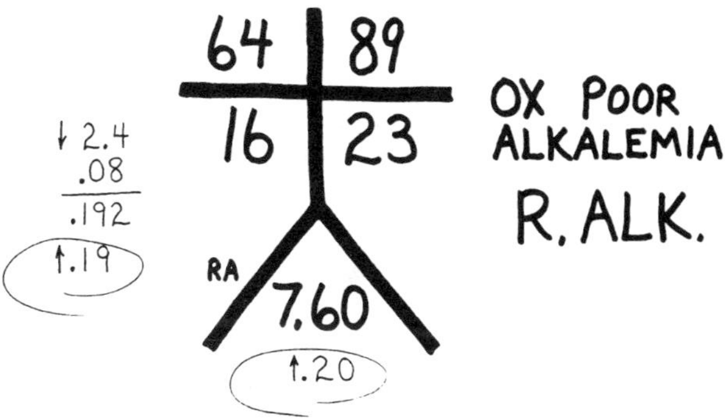

6j. EXAMPLE:

A thirty-two-year-old female is known to be severely allergic to aspirin. She took a new over-the-counter "pain pill." A short time later, she presents with chest pain, dyspnea, wheezing, and light-headedness. She has an audible stridor and diffuse multi-tonal musical wheezing throughout the lungs. The EKG shows global ischemia. Respirations are 42 and blood pressure 84/20. She is on 4 liters O_2 by mask.

Blood gases show a pO_2 of 251.2 and O_2 SAT of 99.9%. The pH is 7.54 with a pCO_2 of 12.0. The bicarb is 14 and BE -4.8. The arterial stick was from the femoral.

This is anaphylaxis. She is having cardiac angina and an acute reactive airway. The airway obstruction is causing her to hyperventilate. The oxygenation is great and she obviously has no CO_2 retention. The metabolic

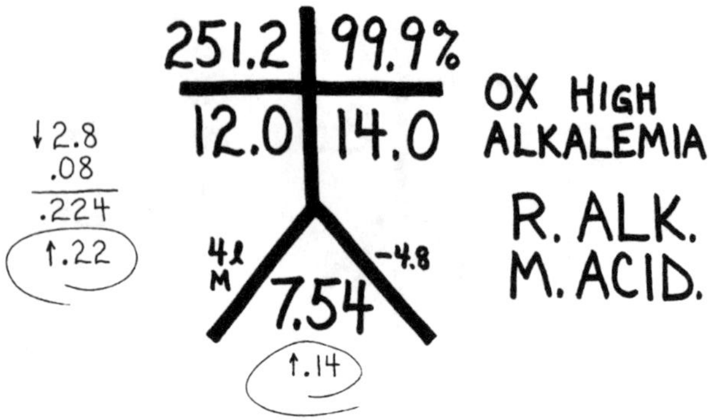

acidosis is secondary to the shock (low tissue perfusion with hypotension.) There are two diagnoses from the ABG standpoint. 1) Hyperventilation and 2) shock. The R. ALK and M. ACID do NOT have much to do with each other in the way of compensation. They each have their own cause. You can't mark the R. ALK as primary since the M. ACID did not come about in order to compensate it.

The next case is the same patient thirty minutes later.

6k. EXAMPLE:

Once the cardiac ischemia was found as a cause of her chest pain, the oxygen was turned up from 4 liters/min to 10—still by mask. Appropriate treatment for anaphylaxis has been given. She is still in severe distress. Respirations are 46.

ABG's now show a pO_2 of 121.8, an O_2 SAT of 98.2%, and a pH of 7.39. The pCO_2 is 25.0 and bicarb 15.2. BE is -7.2.

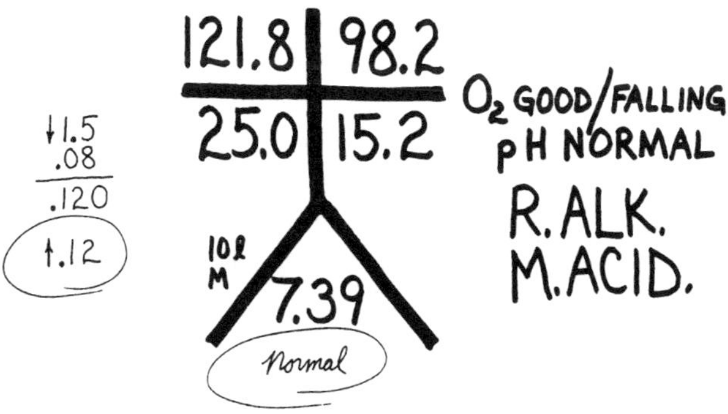

There is no change in diagnoses. I presented this case to show a few hidden dangers. This gal nearly died. Note that in spite of almost doubling the administered O_2, the respiratory rate has climbed and the pO_2 has dropped by more than half. The pCO_2 although still low, has more than doubled. This is a relative hypercarbia since a respiratory rate of 46 should blow the pCO_2 off much better.

This example shows the value of serial ABG determinations. One could easily be fooled by the apparent "good numbers" of the second draw in this case. Don't ignore oxygenation information. Watch for relative hypercarbia. This patient simply "pooped out" by breathing against the reactive airway. She subsequently was placed on a ventilator and recovered fully.

61. EXAMPLE:

A seventy-one-year-old man, a close friend, is dying of emphysema. He is home oxygen dependent at 2 liters per minute. He presents in extreme distress. He wants no intubation nor ventilator support. O_2 is given at 10 liters by mask.

The initial blood gases show a pH of 6.97. The pO_2 is 108.9 and the O_2 SAT 92.5%. The bicarb is 39.0. The pCO_2 is 166.4. BE is 2.4.

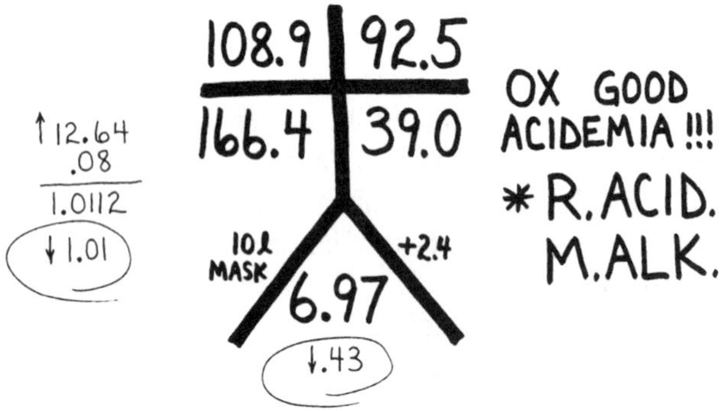

The oxygenation is very good but requires 10 liters of O_2 to attain it. The severe finding is the hypercarbia. It is extreme. The pCO_2 change predicts a pH drop of 1.01, but the actual pH dropped less than half that amount. The metabolic alkalosis is preventing the severe drop and "holding up" the pH. There has been a chronic bicarb retention, telling us that the hypercarbia is long standing (not unusual with emphysema). The pCO_2 of 166.4, however, is nearly a lethal level and is certainly acute. The acidemia is almost incompatible with life. The next example is several hours later.

6m. EXAMPLE:

Hours later the patient in 61 is comatose. The administered oxygen has been increased to 15 liters per minute by cannula. An amp of bicarb has been given. The ABG's now show the pO_2 at 98.3 and O_2 SAT of 89.5. The pH is unchanged at 6.97. The pCO_2 has increased to 194.3. The bicarb is now 45.0 with a BE of 7.1.

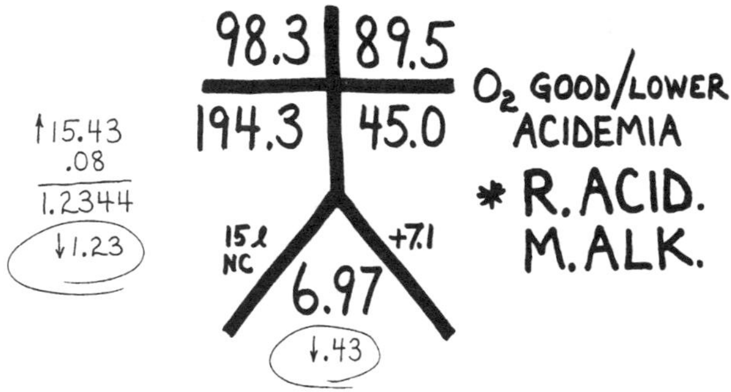

This patient died minutes after this ABG was drawn. With the higher administered oxygen, the pO_2 still dropped somewhat.

Because of the sodium bicarbonate given, the HCO_3 rose from 39 to 45. At the same time, the pCO_2 rose from 166 to 194. The net effect was that the pH remained exactly the same (acid and base both rose equally). The hypercarbia proved lethal and respirations quietly ceased. It is ironic that this man died with a pO_2 of nearly 100.

6n. EXAMPLE:

This case is of a sixty-three-year-old female with longtime chronic lung disease. She presents with an acute exacerbation of respiratory distress. An upper airway infection and mild acute reactive airway change is evident on physical exam.

The blood gases are drawn on room air. Respirations are 46.

The pH is 7.40. Oxygenation shows a pO_2 48.7 with O_2 SAT of 83.2%. The pCO_2 is 51.0. Bicarb is 31.8 and BE +6.2.

The patient is a card-carrying 50-50 club member. The respiratory acidosis predicts a pH drop that isn't seen. The metabolic alkalosis perfectly counters it, giving a normal pH. The next example is two hours after O_2 is given.

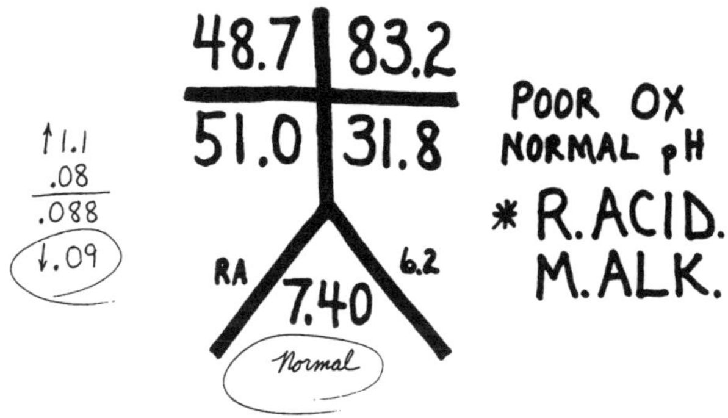

6o. EXAMPLE:

The patient in 6n is given oxygen at 4 liters, having been on room air originally. The patient didn't note any change in her dyspnea. However, the respirations were noted to drop to 28.

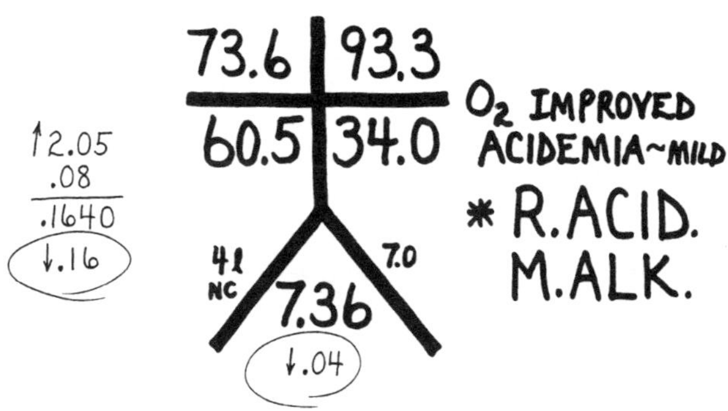

ABG's now show a pO_2 of 73.6 with an O_2 SAT of 93.3%. The pH is 7.36 and pCO_2 60.5. The bicarb is 34.0 with a BE of 7.0.

Note that the patient does not "feel" any change—better or worse—in her dyspnea. The administered oxygen has improved the pO_2 and O_2 SAT, but it has diminished her reflex for breathing and so the respiratory rate has fallen from 46 to 28. This caused a worsening of her CO_2 retention.

This example illustrates the concept of hypoxic drive in chronic lung patients (see COPD/Emphysema in chapter III). A pCO_2 increase of 10 in a non-chronic lung patient would likely provoke dyspnea. Furthermore, the administration of O_2 in a non-chronic lung patient would not elevate pCO_2 in the first place, nor would it be likely to drop respiratory rate.

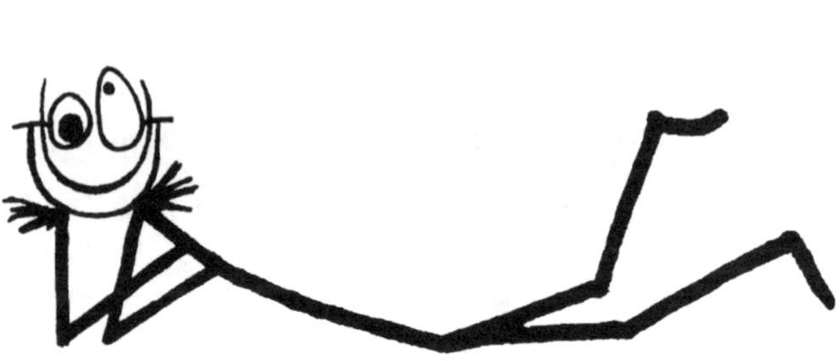

This concludes the examples and so ends the book.

I sincerely hope you are soon a crack "stick 'n study" ABG artist. If not, you will have truly sucker-punched my inner child since on the flip side of the coin wherein it is stamped, "THE STUDENT FAILED TO LEARN" is the ego-stomping inscription, "THE TEACHER FAILED TO TEACH."

May your career be long, your temper longer, and all your arterial samples bright cherry red. If you do have any trouble with "A B GEEZ" in the wee hours of the morning, please feel free to call. My ex-wife's number in Phoenix is 1 (700) 555–1000.